HEART
SOUNDS
AND
MURMURS
ACROSS THE LIFESPAN

HEART SOUNDS AND MURMURS

ACROSS THE LIFESPAN

FOURTH EDITION

Barbara Erickson, PhD, RN, CCRN

Cardiovascular Clinical Nurse Specialist/Research Analyst
Department of Medicine, Research and Education, Inc.
Youngstown, Ohio

With 78 illustrations

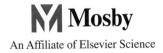
Mosby

An Affiliate of Elsevier Science

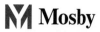 **Mosby**

An Affiliate of Elsevier Science

11830 Westline Industrial Drive
St. Louis, Missouri 63146

NOTICE

Critical care nursing is an ever-changing field. Standard safety precautions must be followed, but as new research and clinical experience broaden our knowledge, changes in treatment and drug therapy may become necessary or appropriate. Readers are advised to check the most current product information provided by the manufacturer of each drug to be administered to verify the recommended dose, the method and duration of administration, and contraindications. It is the responsibility of the licensed prescriber, relying on experience and knowledge of the patient, to determine dosages and the best treatment for each individual patient. Neither the publisher nor the author assumes any liability for any injury and/or damage to persons or property arising from this publication.

The Publisher

Previous editions copyrighted 1987, 1991, 1997

International Stardand Book Numbers
ISBN 0-323-02033-X
ISBN 0-323-02045-3

Publisher: Barbara Nelson Cullen
Editor: Sandra Clark Brown
Associate Developmental Editor: Adrienne Simon
Publishing Services Manager: Deborah Vogel
Project Manager: Mary Drone
Design Manager: Bill Drone
Cover Design: Studio Montage
Cover Art: Getty Images

Printed in the United States of America

Last digit is the print number: 9   8   7   6   5   4   3   2   1

Preface

Cardiac auscultation is perhaps the most basic and effective assessment technique for evaluating the cardiovascular system. The art of cardiac auscultation was almost lost in favor of other procedures, but it has again come into favor with the recent pressure to control medical costs. Cardiac auscultation is inexpensive and quick when compared to the costs of other diagnostic techniques such as ECGs, phonocardiogram, TEE, or cardiac catheterizations. Findings from a thorough cardiac auscultation may be required to justify more expensive tests. Cardiac auscultation is an essential skill to acquire. The information derived from a properly used stethoscope is invaluable. In the hands of an individual prepared to use it, the stethoscope is a cost-effective, cost-containing invaluable instrument.

Proficiency in cardiac auscultation does not come automatically with the acquisition of a quality stethoscope. The most important prerequisite for effective auscultation is a prepared mind. The clinician should be aware of the dynamics of the cardiac cycle during auscultation and integrate each heart sound and murmur heard with a corresponding hemodynamic effect.

The fourth edition of this book expands on the information and interpretation found in the earlier editions to include sounds specific to the pediatric and geriatric populations. Information on common adult abnormalities is also included.

This program is intended for the beginning auscultator who wishes to learn the basics of listening to and interpreting heart sounds. The more advanced auscultator may find the program helpful as a review. The format used is one that has proven successful to the author over many years of teaching heart sounds. Basic information in the text is accompanied by an audio program. By first reading the text and then listening to the audio program, the learner should have the information essential to understanding and recognizing the normal heart sounds and the most common abnormal sounds.

To become clinically proficient in recognizing heart sounds, the learner is advised to continually listen to as many hearts as possible. However good the reproduction of heart sounds on the audio program may be, the program can never replace the experience of listening to actual heart sounds. Please remember that the sounds on the audio program have been distinctly simulated to facilitate learning. Sounds from real hearts are never heard as clearly as those from a simulation.

Most of the audio program was made with a heart sound simulator, using studio recording equipment. Only a few sounds recorded from real hearts have been incorporated into the program.

Barbara Erickson

REVIEWER

Angela J. DiSabatino, RN, MS
Manager, Cardiovascular Research
Christiana Care Health Services, Inc.
Cardiovascular Research Program
Christiana Hospital
Newark, Delaware

Instructions For Use

THE LEARNER IS ADVISED TO:

1. Read the basic information found in the text regarding the sound.
2. Listen to the sound on the accompanying audio program, which should be repeatedly listened to until the learner is able to discern the sound being described. Before proceeding to the next section, the learner must understand and *identify* each sound being described.
3. Listen to the audio program with a stethoscope placed about 4 inches from the speaker. For best results, the audio program should be played on quality equipment. The better the sound transmission of the equipment, the better the learner will be able to hear subtle differences on the heart sound audio program.
4. Listen to real hearts. Repeatedly practice listening to heart sounds to gain proficiency and expertise.
5. Test your knowledge of the content of each chapter by:
   a. Comparing behavioral objectives given at the beginning of each chapter to your abilities on completing the chapter.
   b. Answering self-learning questions at the end of each chapter and checking your answers against those in the answer key.
   c. Listening to the "unknowns" on the audio program at the end of each chapter and checking your answers against those in the answer key.
6. Refer to the audio program when the symbol ⚡ appears in the margin.

Contents

Chapter 3
The Second Heart Sound (S_2), 27

Chapter 4
The Fourth Heart Sound (S_4), 33

Chapter 5
The Third Heart Sound (S_3), 39

Chapter 6
Murmurs—General Information, 44

Chapter 7
Systolic Murmurs, 52

Chapter 8
Diastolic Murmurs, 59

Chapter 9
Sounds Around S$_1$, 65

Chapter 10
Sounds Around S$_2$, 73

Chapter 11
Friction Rubs: Pericardial and Pleural, 81

Chapter 12
Prosthetic Valve Sounds, 87

Chapter 13
Sounds After Heart Surgery and Other Sounds, 95

Chapter 14 ——————————————————
Common Adult Abnormalities, 101

Chapter 15 ——————————————————
Geriatric Heart Sounds, 110

Chapter 16
Introduction to Pediatric Auscultation, 119

Chapter 17
Pediatric Systolic Murmurs, 128

Chapter 18
Pediatric Diastolic Murmurs, 145

Chapter 19
Pediatric Murmurs with Both Systolic and Diastolic Components, 152

Chapter 20
When to Refer, 166

Appendix: Transcript for Audio Program, 171

Bibliography, 184

Glossary, 185

C·H·A·P·T·E·R

1

Introduction

LEARNING OBJECTIVES

After reading this chapter and answering the self-learning questions at the end of the chapter, the learner will be able to:

1. Identify the requirements for adequate cardiac auscultation.
2. Differentiate between the use of the bell and the diaphragm chestpiece of a stethoscope.
3. Identify two basic mechanisms of cardiac sound production.
4. Identify the four basic characteristics of sound.
5. Differentiate between sounds of high frequency and low frequency.
6. Identify three factors that enter into the transmission of sounds.
7. Choose the appropriate area on the chest for auscultation of a selected sound.
8. Differentiate between ventricular systole, ventricular diastole, and atrial systole.
9. Identify the relationship of cardiac sounds to the cardiac cycle.
10. Chart heart sounds using the one-through-six classification scale.

HISTORY

The language of the heart, discerned by cardiac auscultation, is a universal medical language. I was dramatically made aware of this while visiting China, where communications needing no interpretation were those of heart sounds, electrocardiograms, and music. By becoming skillful in listening to and interpreting the language of the heart, you also may join a long line of notable semiologists.

Direct auscultation of the heart was known to Hippocrates (460-377 BC), who may have used heart sounds for diagnostic purposes. William Harvey (1578-1657) seems to have been the first to make specific reference to heart sounds. The use of the ear without mechanical aid was the accepted method of listening to the heart until 1816, when René Laënnec invented the first stethoscope. Laënnec (1781-1826), by discovering and perfecting the acoustic trumpet, became known as the "Father of Auscultation." Laënnec named his auscultatory instrument a "stethoscope" from the Greek word meaning "the spy of the chest." His original instrument, which was a hollow, wooden cylinder, has been repeatedly revised. These revisions have continued to the present, making available a great variety of quality stethoscopes.

However perfect the instrument of auscultation is, the interpretation of the sounds is still its essence. Although Laënnec devoted his life to the semiology of cardiac auscultation, it was a Czech doctor, Joseph Skoda (1805-1881), who first described the cardiac sounds and murmurs. He pinpointed their locations and defined the clinical auscultatory signs that have allowed the diagnosis of cardiac pathologic conditions via auscultation. The learner is advised to mimic Skoda and become proficient in pinpointing the locations of cardiac sounds and murmurs to arrive at a clinical interpretation of their meaning.

REQUIREMENTS FOR AUSCULTATION

Auscultation must not be performed as an isolated event. The total cardiovascular physical examination includes five important parts: (1) examination of the arterial pulse and blood pressure, (2) inspection of the jugular venous pulse, (3) inspection of the precordium, (4) palpation of the precordium, and (5) auscultation. Each of these parts is important, although only auscultation is discussed in this book.

One of the first things to consider when undertaking auscultation of the heart is the necessity to:

1. Use a quiet, well-lit, warm room. To facilitate hearing the heart sounds, ambient noise in the room should be eliminated as much

as possible. This means that room doors are closed, equipment such as radios and televisions are turned off, and conversations are stopped. Unfortunately, a quiet room may be one of the hardest elements to achieve. The room needs to be well lit so that the inspection aspect of cardiac examination may be done. Many of the heart sounds can be seen and felt, as well as heard. A warm room helps keep the patient from shivering, thus causing extraneous sounds under the chestpiece of the stethoscope.

2. Have the patient properly disrobed. The stethoscope should always be placed in direct contact with the chest wall. Most abnormal sounds cannot be heard through clothing because they are lower in frequency and softer than normal heart sounds. Also, listening through clothing will produce sound distortions caused by the stethoscope rubbing against the clothing.

3. Examine the patient in three positions—sitting, supine, and left lateral recumbent (Figure 1-1). Listening with the patient in various positions will bring out certain heart sounds, especially some abnormal ones. For instance, the third heart sound (S_3) may be brought out by having the patient turn to the left lateral recumbent position.

4. Examine the patient from his or her right side. Being on the patient's right side forces the examiner to reach across the chest to listen to the heart. This stretches out the tubing of the stethoscope and decreases the likelihood of extraneous sounds caused by the tubing hitting objects (e.g., chest wall, side rails).

5. Use a stethoscope with a bell and diaphragm chestpiece or one with characteristics of both bell and diaphragm. Traditionally, a stethoscope with both a bell and a diaphragm was essential for

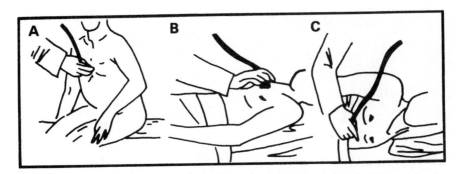

Figure 1-1   Basic positions for cardiac auscultation. **A,** Sitting. **B,** Supine. **C,** Left lateral recumbent. (Reproduced with permission from Caccamo L, Erickson B: *Cardiac auscultation*, Youngstown, Ohio, 1975, St. Elizabeth's Hospital Medical Center.)

complete cardiac auscultation. However, recent technology has provided a stethoscope with only one chestpiece capable of differentiating low-frequency from high-frequency sounds, depending on the pressure applied to the chestpiece. When the chestpiece is used with light pressure, the low-frequency sounds dominate; used with firm pressure, the high-frequency sounds are accentuated. Regardless of the technical advances, the traditional principles still apply and therefore are used in this book.

  a. Using the bell: When the bell is held lightly (leaving no after-imprint on the chest), it picks up low-frequency sounds. Pressure on the bell causes the skin to be pulled tautly over the bottom of the bell, changing the bell to a diaphragm (Figure 1-2).

  b. Using the diaphragm: When the diaphragm is applied firmly (leaving an after-imprint), it picks up high-frequency sounds.

  c. Differentiating frequencies: The frequency of a sound is readily identified by noting with which chestpiece of the stethoscope the sound is best heard. A sound best heard or only heard with the bell held lightly is of low frequency. A sound best heard with the bell applied firmly or with a diaphragm is of high frequency. This simple maneuver of listening to a sound with the bell held lightly and then applied firmly permits you to determine the frequency of the sound to which you are listening. This is an important point to remember.

6. Listen to each area of auscultation. Listen to each of the following areas, using first the diaphragm and then the bell (Figure 1-3).

  a. Left lateral sternal border (LLSB) (also known as *lower left sternal border*): This is the fourth intercostal space (4 ICS) to the left of

A 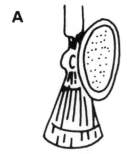 **B**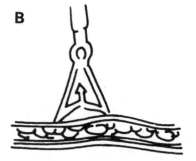

Figure 1-2   Using the chestpiece. **A,** *Lightly* applied to skin (no after-imprint is left) transmits *low*-frequency sounds. **B,** *Firmly* applied to skin (leaves an after-imprint) with skin pulled tautly over the bottom of the bell changes it into a diaphragm and transmits *high*-frequency sounds. (Modified with permission from Caccamo L, Erickson B: *Cardiac auscultation*, Youngstown, Ohio, 1975, St. Elizabeth's Hospital Medical Center.)

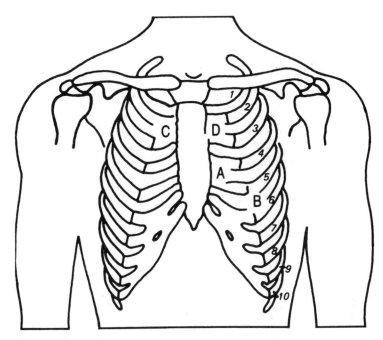

Figure 1-3   Sites for auscultation. **A,** *Left lateral sternal border* (sounds from tricuspid valve and right side of heart heard best). **B,** *Apex* (sounds from mitral valve and left side of heart heard best). **C,** *Base right* (sounds from aortic valve heard best). **D,** *Base left* (sounds from pulmonic valve heard best).

     the sternum. Sounds from the tricuspid valve and right heart are best heard.

  b. Apex: This is the fifth intercostal space (5 ICS) in the midclavicular line. Sounds from the mitral valve and left heart are best heard.

  c. Base right (previously known as *aortic area*): This is the second intercostal space (2 ICS) to the right of the sternum. Sounds from the aortic valve are best heard.

  d. Base left (previously known as *pulmonic area*): This is the second intercostal space (2 ICS) to the left of the sternum. Sounds from the pulmonic valve are best heard.

7. Use a sequence for auscultation. Each time you listen to a heart, begin at the same cardiac area. Listen to all of the four areas just mentioned, using the same order each time. This will help you establish a routine for yourself; you will "automatically" listen to all four areas each time you auscultate a heart. The order in which you listen is an individual preference. If you already have established such a personal preference, do not feel obliged to change it. If you

are suspicious that aortic regurgitation is present, there is a fifth area at which you should listen. This is Erb's point—the third intercostal space (3 ICS) to the left of the sternum.

8. Use selective listening. Listen to one thing at a time. When listening to the first heart sound (S_1), do not be concerned about the second heart sound (S_2). If listening to sounds in systole, do not be concerned about the sounds in diastole. With experience you will be able to rapidly assess the total heart sounds. Selective listening is a skill that is honed with practice. You may improve this skill by picking out a favorite instrument in a musical arrangement or listening for the ticking of a clock or other repetitive noise in your daily environment. The skill of selective listening is transferable from one situation to another.

CARDIAC CYCLE

The cardiac cycle consists of two periods: one of contraction (systole) and one of relaxation (diastole). During systole, the heart chambers eject blood; during diastole, the heart chambers fill with blood. These events are represented on pressure curves (Figure 1-4).

Ventricular systole follows closure of the mitral and tricuspid valves. This systolic period is divided into two phases:

1. The first part of the systolic period has two subdivisions.
   a. This period begins with the first initial rise in ventricular pressure after the closure of the mitral and tricuspid valves. It is known also as the *isovolumic contraction phase.*
   b. It is followed by rapid ventricular ejection, which occurs when ventricular pressure exceeds the pressure in the aorta and the pulmonary artery. This forces the aortic and pulmonic valves to open, causing blood to be rapidly ejected from the ventricles.
2. During the latter part of ventricular systole, ventricular pressure falls and reduced ventricular ejection occurs. This period lasts until ventricular ejection stops and ventricular diastole begins.

Ventricular diastole follows closure of the aortic and pulmonic valves. This diastolic period is divided into three phases:

1. The first third of the diastolic period has two subdivisions.
   a. Initially in this period no blood enters the ventricles; therefore they do not increase in volume. This is known also as the *isovolumic relaxation phase.*
   b. When atrial pressure exceeds ventricular pressure, the mitral and tricuspid valves open and blood rapidly enters the ventricles. This is known also as the *rapid filling phase.*

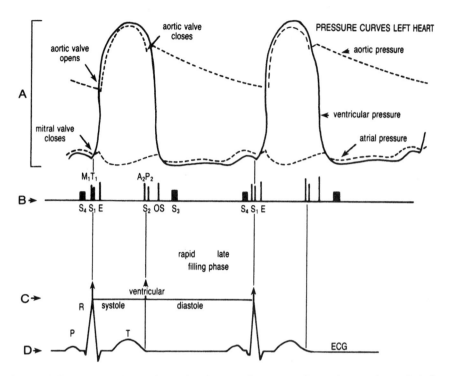

Figure 1-4   Time relationships of various cardiac events. *From the top down:* **A,** Left heart pressure curves—aortic, ventricular, and atrial. **B,** Heart sounds—normal (S_1: made of M_1 and T_1 closure; S_2: made of A_2 and P_2 closure) and extra (S_4, ejection [E], opening snap [OS], and S_3). **C,** Cardiac cycle—ventricular systole and diastole. **D,** Electrocardiogram (ECG).

2. During the middle third of the diastolic period, there is almost no inflow into the ventricles. This is the period during which both the atria and the ventricles are relaxed.
3. During the last third of the diastolic period, atrial contraction or "atrial kick" occurs and the remaining blood is squeezed from the atria. This is known also as the *late filling phase.*

Atrial systole occurs during the last third of ventricular diastole. Atrial systole may contribute 20% to 25% to ventricular filling. The contribution is less at faster heart rates (100 beats/min or more).

CARDIAC SOUND-CYCLE RELATIONSHIP

Cardiac sounds are named according to their sequence of occurrence and are produced at specific points in the cardiac cycle. The initial sound heard is the first heart sound, or S_1. It occurs at the beginning of ventricular systole when ventricular volume is maximal. The sound occurring at the end of ventricular systole is the second heart sound, or S_2. The period between S_1 and S_2 represents ventricular systole; the period following S_2 and the next S_1 represents ventricular diastole (see Figure 1-4).

CARDIAC VALVE AREAS

Sounds from the heart valves (mitral, tricuspid, aortic, and pulmonic) are heard at specific areas on the chest. As discussed:
1. Mitral valve sounds and other left heart sounds are best heard at the apex.
2. Tricuspid valve sounds and other right heart sounds are best heard at the LLSB.
3. Aortic valve sounds are best heard at base right.
4. Pulmonic valve sounds are best heard at base left.

The anatomic location of the valve and the auscultatory area (area best heard) are not synonymous (see Figure 6-1).

The amount of energy behind the heart sound's production is a contributory factor behind its auscultatory area. Because left heart sounds have more energy behind their productions, they are audible anywhere on the precordium. Right heart sounds, with less energy behind their productions, usually are best heard at only one area—the site to which they radiate.

CARDIAC SOUND PRODUCTION

Cardiac sound production results from at least two basic mechanisms:
1. The sudden acceleration or deceleration of blood, which is influenced mainly by:
   a. The opening and closing of heart valves
   b. Sudden tension of intracardiac structures (e.g., chordae tendineae, papillary muscles, chamber walls)
2. Turbulent blood flow produced when anatomically there is one of the following:
   a. Unilateral protrusion into the bloodstream
   b. Circumferential narrowing
   c. Flow into a distal chamber of larger diameter than the proximal chamber
   d. Flow into a distal chamber of smaller diameter than the proximal chamber
   e. High flow rates

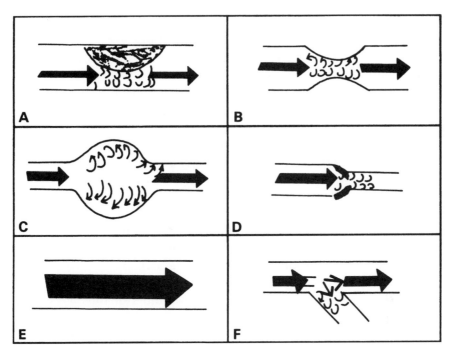

Figure 1-5   Factors producing turbulence. **A,** Unilateral protrusion into the bloodstream. **B,** Circumferential narrowing. **C,** Distal chamber larger than proximal one. **D,** Distal chamber smaller than proximal one. **E,** High flow rates. **F,** Abnormal communications (e.g., ventricular septal defect [VSD]).

     f. Abnormal communications (e.g., ventricular septal defect, atrial septal defect)

These conditions can cause eddies in the vascular system and produce audible vibrations (Figure 1-5).

CHARACTERISTICS OF SOUND

Four basic characteristics of sound must be considered: (1) frequency, (2) intensity, (3) quality, and (4) duration.

   1. Frequency is the number of wave cycles generated per second by a vibrating body. It is vibratory movement of an object in motion that initiates the sound-wave cycles that can be discerned with the stethoscope. Frequency determines pitch—a subjective sensation that indicates to the listener whether the tone is high or low on a musical scale.

     a. High frequency: The greater the number of wave cycles per second, the higher the frequency and the pitch. High-frequency sounds are best heard with the diaphragm of the stethoscope applied firmly so that an after-imprint is seen on the chest.

   b. Low frequency: The fewer the number of wave cycles per second, the lower the frequency and pitch. Low-frequency sounds are best heard with the bell of the stethoscope held lightly so that no after-imprint is seen on the chest.

2. Intensity is related to the height of the sound wave produced by a vibrating object. Intensity determines the loudness of the perceived sound. High-amplitude waves are produced when an object vibrates with great energy; they are heard as loud sounds. Low-amplitude waves occur when an object vibrates with low energy; they are heard as soft sounds.

3. Quality distinguishes two sounds with equal degrees of frequency and intensity but that come from a different source (piano from violin, or heart sounds from breath sounds).

4. Duration is the length of time the sound lasts. Heart sounds (S_1 and S_2) are of short duration. Cardiac murmurs or rubs are of long duration.

These four characteristics should be considered when listening to the heart. Only with experience can the subtleties of sound characteristics be appreciated—much as the quiet stirring of a restless child awakens only its mother while others sleep.

SOUND TRANSMISSION

Three factors enter into how well a sound is transmitted from its source to the auscultator's ears: (1) the type of substance through which it travels, (2) the quality of the stethoscope, and (3) the human ear.

1. Types of substances
   a. Bone is an excellent transmitter of sound.
   b. Blood and muscle are fair transmitters.
   c. Air is a poor transmitter. Therefore the lung, which is normally filled with air, is a poor transmitter of sound. During cardiac auscultation, the heart sounds are best heard in individuals with thin chests because the sounds are being transmitted primarily by blood, muscle, or bone. Cardiac auscultation is more difficult in individuals with thick chests. Obesity, or increased adipose tissue, will decrease sound transmission, as will conditions that cause increased anterior-posterior (A-P) diameter from air-trapping (chronic obstructive lung disease).

2. The stethoscope
   The stethoscope chosen must be of good quality and have both a

bell and a diaphragm chestpiece or one that combines the bell and diaphragm modes into a single-side chestpiece. The quality of the sound transmitted is affected by the design and structural factors of the stethoscope. The tubing of the stethoscope must permit the heart sounds to be transmitted to the ears without loss of quality and without the introduction of ambient noises from the environment. Whether to use a scope with a double or single tube is debatable. Theoretically, sound transmission is better with the double tube, although opinions differ on this. The single-tube stethoscope has certain mechanical advantages: less bulk, less ambient noise from the tubes rubbing on each other, and a smaller surface to pick up outside noise. The length of the tubing should be as short as feasible for the clinical situation in which it is used routinely. Regardless of the type of stethoscope chosen, the earpieces must fit the examiner's ear canal comfortably; they should be neither too tight nor too loose. Very small ear tips penetrate deeply into the canals, actually causing pain; very large tips may occlude the canals. Neither fit facilitates auscultation.

Electronic or amplifying stethoscopes are now available that provide amplification up to 18 times greater than the finest conventional stethoscope. Some clinicians may find this amplification necessary and of value. However, amplified heart sounds may be unlike the way they ordinarily are heard with the binaural stethoscope. This may cause difficulty in interpreting the sounds and in differentiating the ambient noises that may be inherent in the amplified instrument from normal or abnormal heart sounds.

A quality stethoscope should provide you with many years of service if you provide reasonable care. Stethoscopes should always be cleaned between patients, using the manufacturer's recommended method such as soap and water or alcohol. If sterilization is required, gas sterilization may be necessary. It is not advisable to soak the stethoscope in any liquid or to subject it to steam sterilization. Extreme heat or cold, solvents, and oils may damage your stethoscope. Always ensure your stethoscope's safety. When feasible, I prefer to carry mine in a lab coat pocket. When left unattended in a clinical area, a quality stethoscope frequently will disappear.

Regardless of the stethoscope chosen, the most important part is that between the two earpieces. A quality stethoscope in the hands of an individual prepared to use it is an invaluable instrument.

3. The human ear

Individuals differ in their ability to hear. The normal human ear is capable of perceiving sounds with a frequency of 20 to 20,000 cycles/second and duration of as little as 0.02 second. The audible components of heart sounds and murmurs are in the frequency range between 30 to 250 cycles/second. Because of the peculiarities of the human ear, high-frequency sounds may seem louder than a low-frequency sound of equal intensity. Also, very loud sounds may momentarily deafen. Therefore the auscultator may have trouble hearing a soft sound that immediately follows a loud sound. High-frequency perception decreases with age, but this should not interfere with cardiac auscultation because heart sounds are in the lower-frequency range of the hearing capability of the ear. This means that the ability to hear heart sounds should improve with age.

CLASSIFICATION OF SOUNDS AND MURMURS

Sounds and murmurs may be classified, or graded, on a one-through-six scale:

1. Not audible during the first few seconds of auscultation; heard after listener tunes in
2. Heard immediately, but faint
3. Loud but without a thrust or thrill
4. Loud with a thrust or thrill
5. Loud with a thrust or thrill and audible with the chestpiece tilted on the chest
6. Loud with a thrust or thrill and audible with the chestpiece just off the chest wall

"Thrust" is an intermittent, palpable (sometimes even visible) sensation at the site being auscultated. This is the sensation felt when palpating the point of maximal impulse at the apex of the heart. "Thrill" is a continuous palpable sensation comparable to the vibration felt when a cat purrs.

To chart a sound or murmur, a fraction is used (3/6 or III/VI). The numerator of the fraction indicates where the sound being described fits into the classification system. The denominator indicates the total number of parts in the classification. Therefore a sound described as a "3/6" would be one that is loud but without a thrust or thrill (as indicated by the numerator "3"). It is being described in a classification system with six parts (as indicated by the denominator "6").

CHARTING HEART SOUNDS

Charting heart sounds includes a description of what is heard at each of the four basic auscultatory sites. Included in the description are the sound characteristics of frequency, intensity, quality, and duration. In addition, the charting should include:

1. Area of auscultation—LLSB, apex, base right, base left
2. Heart rate
3. Patient's position—e.g., supine, sitting, left lateral recumbent
4. Description of S_1 and S_2
5. Presence of other sounds—splits, ejection sounds, clicks, S_3, S_4
6. Presence of murmurs—noting:
   a. Location of valve area where murmur is best heard
   b. Loudness (intensity) by using one-through-six classification
   c. Frequency (pitch)—low, medium, or high
   d. Quality—blowing, harsh or rough, or rumble
   e. Timing—systolic or diastolic
   f. Finer timing—early, mid, late, or pan
   g. Radiation—other locations murmur is heard
   h. Increase or decrease of murmur with respiration, position, special maneuvers, or drugs
7. The type of stethoscope chestpiece used—bell or diaphragm
8. The effect of respiration (e.g., inspiration or expiration) or other maneuvers (e.g., standing, squatting, Valsalva)

The auscultogram, a graphic method of charting heart sounds, is one of the easiest methods to use. The auscultogram provides an easy means of drawing what is heard during cardiac auscultation. The auscultogram includes:

1. A drawing of the chest with the four basic auscultatory sites marked
2. Blank blocks drawn one on top of the other, six blocks high; each block represents one classification in the grading system, with one being the bottom block and six being the top block
3. S_1 and S_2 represented by vertical lines drawn in the blank blocks to indicate the intensity of the sounds
4. S_3, S_4, splits, clicks, and ejection sounds if heard
5. Murmurs, which are represented by sine waves
   a. Widely spaced for low frequency
   b. Close picket-fence lines for high frequency

The loudness is represented by the height of the wave on a one-through-six scale (Figure 1-6).

Name _____ Date _____

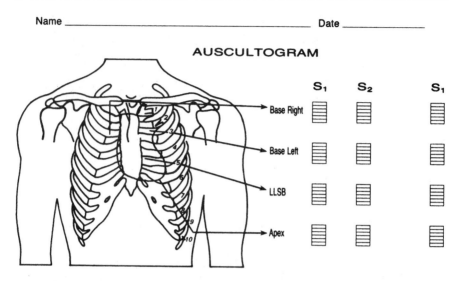

AUSCULTOGRAM

Indicate the loudness of the S_1 and S_2 at each of the auscultatory sites by drawing vertical lines to the appropriate height in the blank blocks using the one-through-six scale:

(Each block represents one classification in the grading system.
"1" being the bottom block and "6" being the top block.)

1. Not audible during the first few seconds of auscultation.
2. Heard immediately but faint.
3. Loud but without a thrust or thrill.*
4. Loud but with a thrust or thrill.
5. Loud with a thrust or thrill and audible with the chestpiece tilted on the chest.
6. Loud with a thrust or thrill and audible with chestpiece just off the chest wall.

*"Thrill" is a *continuous* palpable sensation comparable to the vibration felt when a cat purrs; "thrust" is an *intermittent* palpable, sometimes even visible, sensation at the site being auscultated.

Draw in extra sound (i.e., S_3, S_4, ejection [E], or clicks [C]) as indicated.

Draw murmurs in the appropriate cycle.

Use the following sine waves to indicate the frequency/quality:

High Frequency = ｌｕｌｌｌｌｌｌｌｕｌｌｌｌｌｌ
(Blowing)

Low Frequency = ᴧᴧᴧᴧᴧᴧᴧᴧ
(Rumbling)

Mixture = ᴧﻭﻭﻭﻭﻭﻭﻭ

Using the one-through-six scale indicate loudness of murmur by drawing sine wave to height comparable to the loudness of the murmur.

Figure 1-6   An auscultogram—a graphic method recording heart sounds and murmurs. *LLSB,* Left lateral sternal border (also known as *lower left sternal border*).

MIMICKING SOUNDS

The quality of cardiac sounds can be captured only by the human ear. Phonocardiography produces visual records but not sound. Trying to appreciate heart sounds by looking at a phonocardiogram would be like trying to appreciate a symphony by merely reading the score. The sounds are transcribed, but the music is lost.

A vocabulary that translates the cardiac sounds into spoken syllables has been developed. The normal heart cycle produces a two-sound cadence that can be simulated by the syllables "lub" and "dub." The prefix "l" is used to represent S_1—"lub"; the prefix "d" is used to represent S_2—"dub." Extra sounds such as S_3, S_4, clicks, and snaps are represented by the prefix "b." The intensity of the sounds is represented as follows:

	S_1	S_2	Extra sounds
1. Faint sounds	"le"	"de"	"be"
2. Normal sounds	"lub"	"dub"	"bub"
3. Loud sounds	"lup"	"dup"	"bup"
4. Very loud sounds	"lupp"	"dupp"	"bupp"

The cadence for a normal S_4 S_1 S_2 would be mimicked by syllables "bub" "lub" "dub." The cadence for a soft S_4 followed by a normal S_1 S_2 would be vocalized as "be" "lub" "dub"; a normal S_1 and S_2 with a loud S_3 would be vocalized as "lub" "dub" "bup."

SELF-LEARNING QUESTIONS

Select the letter of the correct response, or provide requested information. Compare your answers with the answer key at the end of the chapter. Reread the chapter as needed to achieve mastery of the content.

1. Name five of the eight requirements for adequate cardiac auscultation.
   a.
   b.
   c.
   d.
   e.

2. Cardiac sounds and murmurs of low frequency can be best heard by using:
   a. a diaphragm chestpiece
   b. a monaural scope
   c. a bell chestpiece
   d. either a bell or a diaphragm chestpiece

3. The two basic mechanisms of cardiac sound production are:
   a.
   b.

4. The number of wave cycles generated per second by a vibrating body is
   a description of the sound characteristic of:
   a. quality   **b.** intensity
   c. frequency   **d.** duration

5. The best type of substance for transmitting sound is:
   a. blood   **b.** fat
   c. air   **d.** bone

6. The frequency perception that is decreased with aging is:
   a. low   **b.** medium
   c. high   **d.** none

7. At which area of the chest would mitral or left heart sounds be best
   heard?
   a. left lateral sternal border   **b.** apex
   c. base right   **d.** base left

8. The rapid filling phase, when the mitral and tricuspid valves open and
   blood rapidly enters the ventricles, is a part of:
   a. atrial systole   **b.** atrial diastole
   c. ventricular systole   **d.** ventricular diastole

9. The cardiac sound that occurs at the beginning of ventricular systole
   when ventricular volume is maximal is called the:
   a. first sound (S_1) **b.** second sound (S_2)
   c. third sound (S_3) **d.** fourth sound (S_4)

10. Indicate the graphic representation of a cardiac sound that is loud
    without a thrill by drawing lines at the appropriate height in the
    following box.

ANSWERS TO SELF-LEARNING QUESTIONS

1. Any five:
   —A quiet, well-lit, warm room
   —A properly disrobed patient
   —Examine in three positions—sitting, supine, and left lateral recumbent
   —Use a stethoscope with a bell and diaphragm chestpiece
   —Listen to at least four basic areas
   —Use a sequence for auscultation
   —Use selective listening
   —Examine patient from right side

2. c

3. —The sudden acceleration or deceleration of blood
   —Turbulent blood flow

4. c

5. d

6. c

7. b

8. d

9. a

10.

C·H·A·P·T·E·R

2

The First Heart Sound (S$_1$)

LEARNING OBJECTIVES

After reading this chapter, listening to the accompanying audio program, answering the self-learning questions at the end of the chapter, and listening to the "unknowns" on the audio program, the learner will be able to:

1. Identify the classical theory behind the production of the S$_1$.
2. Differentiate between a single S$_1$ and a normal split S$_1$.
3. Recognize a normal S$_1$ at the various auscultatory sites.
4. Identify the physiological factors that affect the intensity of S$_1$.
5. Identify methods of differentiating S$_1$ from S$_2$.

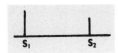

COMPONENTS OF S₁

The classical and generally accepted theory for the production of S₁ is that S₁ is associated with the closure of the mitral (M₁) and tricuspid (T₁) valves. The latest theory indicates that it is the change in the rate of pressure rise in the ventricles, causing sudden tension of intracardiac structures, which contributes to the first heart sound production. The classical theory, although not entirely true, is "simple" and easily correlated with clinical findings and therefore is used for the text. Because S₁ is caused by the closure of two separate valves, both must be considered when listening to it.

M₁ is the first audible component of S₁. This component normally occurs before T₁. (Left-sided mechanical events occur before right-sided mechanical events.) M₁ occurs just after the mitral valve closes. This occurs approximately 0.02 to 0.03 second after left ventricular pressure equals left atrial pressure. M₁ is of slightly higher intensity and frequency than T₁ and is discernible at all the auscultatory sites but is best heard at the apex. Because it is a high-frequency sound, it is best heard with the diaphragm pressed firmly.

T₁ is the second component of S₁. It normally follows M₁ just after the tricuspid valve closes. Because less energy is behind the production of this sound, it may be heard only at the left lateral sternal border (LLSB), the area to which T₁ radiates or is best heard. Because it is a high-frequency sound, it is best heard with the diaphragm applied firmly.

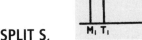

SPLIT S₁

When both components that make S₁ (M₁ and T₁) are separately distinguishable, it is known as a *split*. In a normal split S₁, the components making the sound are 0.02 second apart (Figure 2-1).

The separation between sounds must be at least 0.02 second or greater for the human ear to hear two definite sounds. Because the normal distance between M₁ and T₁ is *only* 0.02 second, a normal split S₁ may be difficult to hear. The ear may perceive it as "slurred" or "fuzzy" and not two separate sounds.

 Listen now to an S₁ that is split at various distances. The initial split will be 0.08 second—the ear will hear two definite sounds. Gradually the interval of the split decreases—0.06 second; then 0.04 second; then 0.02 second (the duration of the normal split S₁).

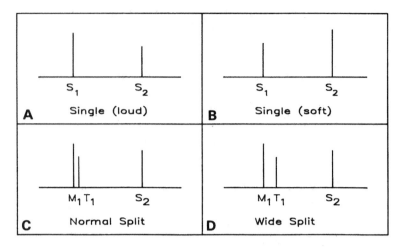

Figure 2-1   Splitting of the first heart sound (S_1). **A,** Single first sound (S_1) louder than the second (S_2). **B,** Single S_1 softer than S_2. **C,** Normal split first sound (M_1T_1) 0.02 second. **D,** Wide split first sound (M_1T_1) 0.04 second. (Reproduced with permission from Caccamo L, Erickson B: *Cardiac auscultation,* Youngstown, Ohio, 1975, St. Elizabeth's Hospital Medical Center.)

Practice listening until you perceive the difference between a single S_1 (only one component audible) and a split S_1 (both components audible).

In a normal heart the split S_1 may be audible only when listening over the area to which the softer tricuspid component radiates—the LLSB. Although a split S_1 is commonly heard in children, it is heard in only about half of normal adults. To be considered a normal split S_1, M_1 and T_1 must be of high frequency and heard close together—0.02 second apart. The split is not affected markedly by respiration. When audible, it is heard consistently.

 Listen now to a normal S_1 at the various sites:
1. LLSB—split or single S_1 heard
2. Apex—single S_1 heard
3. Base right—single S_1 heard
4. Base left—single S_1 heard

INTENSITY OF FIRST SOUND (S_1)

The intensity, or loudness, of S_1 also changes, depending on the site auscultated. S_1 always is slightly louder than S_2 at either the LLSB or the apex. (The M_1 component of the first sound is best heard at the apex; the T_1 component of the first sound is best heard at the LLSB.) S_1 is softer than the second sound (S_2) at either base left or base right. (The aortic [A_1] component of the S_2 is best heard at base right; the pulmonic [P_1] component of S_2 is best heard at base left.)

When a loud sound is followed by a soft sound, the ear perceives the sound as coming down a musical scale. When a soft sound is followed by a loud sound, the ear perceives the sound as going up a musical scale.

 Listen to the normal S_1 at the various sites:

    1. LLSB—S_1 slightly louder than S_2
    2. Apex—S_1 slightly louder than S_2
    3. Base right—S_1 slightly softer than S_2

When listening to a normal S_1, the following occurs at each specified site:

    1. LLSB—single S_1 or split S_1 louder than S_2
    2. Apex—single S_1 louder than S_2
    3. Base right—single S_1 softer than S_2
    4. Base left—single S_1 softer than S_2

The intensity of S_1 may be affected by the following physiological factors as well:

1. The anatomy of the chest. Sounds are easier to hear and therefore louder in patients with thin chests. Sounds are harder to hear and therefore softer in patients with thick chests.
2. The vigor of ventricular contraction. Sounds are louder when more energy is behind their production, as occurs with a tachycardia. Sounds are softer when less energy is behind their production, as occurs with heart muscle damage (myocardial infarction).
3. Valve position at the onset of ventricular contraction. If the valve leaflets are wide open when they are forced closed, as occurs with a short PR interval (from onset of the P wave to onset of the QRS or R wave—normally 0.12 to 0.20 second), the resulting sound is loud. If the valve leaflets are almost shut when they are forced closed, as occurs with a long PR interval, the resulting sound is soft.
4. Pathological alteration of the valve structure (stiffness of the valve). If the valve orifice is closed and fixed, a loud sound may be heard. If the valve orifice is open and fixed, a soft sound may be heard.

For a synopsis of the physiological factors that vary the intensity of S_1 and the resultant type of sound, see Table 2-1.

TABLE 2-1
Physiological Factors that Vary First Heart Sound (S₁) Intensity

Physiological Factors	Loud S₁	Soft S₁	Variable S₁
1. Anatomy of chest	Thin chest	Emphysema (barrel chest) Obesity Pericardial effusion Edema of chest wall	
2. Vigor of ventricular contraction	Tachycardia: • Exercise • Emotion • Hyperthyroid • Fever Systemic hypertension	Extensive muscle damage (e.g., myocardial infarction)	
3. Valve position at onset of ventricular contraction when valve mobile	Short PR interval (except WPW) when valve wide open with wide arc of closure ASD when tricuspid wide open because of volume load	Long PR interval when valve almost closed with narrow arc at closure	Mobitz I (regular sequential variability of sound) Atrial fibrillation CBH A-V dissociation (irregular variability of sound)
4. Pathological alteration of the valve structure (STIFF)	Mitral stenosis,* which keeps orifice closed and fixed	Mitral regurgitation, which keeps valve open and fixed	

Modified with permission from Caccamo L, Erickson B: *Cardiac auscultation*, Youngstown, Ohio, 1975, St. Elizabeth Hospital Medical Center.
*When the first sound is *loud* and the heart rate is normal, *think mitral stenosis*.
WPW, Wolff-Parkinson-White syndrome; *ASD*, atrial septal defect; *CHB*, complete heart block; *A-V*, atrial-ventricular.

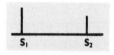

DIFFERENTIATING S₁ FROM S₂

When listening to the normal heart sounds, S₁ and S₂, it is important to be able to know which sound is the first and which is the second. The following suggestions will help make this differentiation.

At a heart rate of 80 beats/minute or less, S₁ follows the longer pause. (The time between S₁ and S₂ [systole] is shorter than the time between S₂ and the next S_1 [diastole].) At a heart rate of more than 80 beats/minute, the diastolic period shortens, becoming equal to systole, and other methods are needed to determine which sound is the first.

In a normal heart, S_2 is always loudest at the base. Therefore listen at the base and determine which of the sounds is the loudest—this is S_2. Then gradually move the stethoscope from the base to the LLSB, keeping in mind which sound is S_1. In this "inching" maneuver, the stethoscope is moved from an area where the sounds are clear to an area where they are not clear. It is a useful technique when multiple or unclear sounds confuse the listener.

Another method of differentiating S_1 from S_2, especially in an individual with a rapid heart rate, is to watch your stethoscope while auscultating. The stethoscope may move outward when placed at the point of maximal impulse (PMI), and the sound heard simultaneously with this outward thrust is S_1.

S_1 also can be timed by simultaneously feeling the carotid pulse while listening to the heart. The sound heard when the carotid is felt is S_1. (Peripheral pulses cannot be used for timing cardiac sounds because time lag is too great between ventricular systole and the palpated peripheral pulse.)

A synopsis of the methods of differentiating S_1 from S_2 is depicted in the algorithm of Figure 2-2.

A big disadvantage of listening to heart sounds on an audio program is that the physiological factor (carotid pulse) that aids in sound differentiation is absent. Therefore it may be more difficult to discern S_1

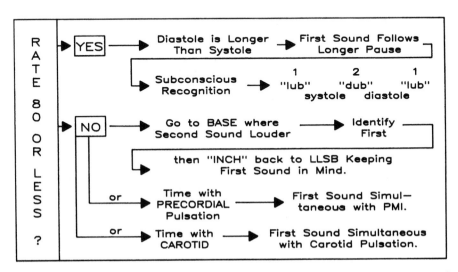

Figure 2-2   Algorithm for differentiating the first heart sound (S_1) from the second heart sound (S_2). (Reproduced with permission from Caccamo L, Erickson B: *Cardiac auscultation*, Youngstown, Ohio, 1975, St. Elizabeth's Hospital Medical Center.)

from S_2. To make it easier for the learner to identify S_1, the rate of the sounds simulated will be 60 beats/minute unless otherwise indicated.

CLINICAL CORRELATION

After gaining confidence in your ability to identify the first heart sound (S_1), hone your ability by listening to as many real hearts as possible. Listen to the thin and the obese and to adults and children, if possible. Note the similarities and differences. Attempt to distinguish a single S_1 from a split S_1. Note the difference in intensity, depending on the site auscultated. Can you differentiate S_1 from S_2 using the physiological factor (carotid pulse) available? Be selective, and listen only to the S_1. The other sounds can be ignored for now. Practice recording the S_1 on an auscultogram.

In listening to patients with fever, anemia, or aortic insufficiency, contractility of the heart is increased and the S_1 will be loud. It is loud also in mitral stenosis or when the heart expels blood against increased resistance, as in systemic hypertension. Listen carefully to S_1 in patients with these findings to see whether you can appreciate a louder-than-normal S_1.

As noted previously, the intensity of S_1 is affected by valve position at the onset of ventricular contraction. Thus a loud S_1 is heard with a short PR interval; a soft S_1 is heard with a long PR interval. Considering the intensity of the first heart sound and the regularity of the cardiac rhythm, the various degrees of heart blocks can be identified by using a stethoscope.

1. First-degree A-V block with prolonged PR interval
   a. S_1 softer than normal
   b. Rhythm regular
2. Second-degree A-V block
   a. Mobitz I (Wenckebach)
      (1) S_1 progressively softens with gradual prolongation of PR interval
      (2) Pause in rhythm at dropped beat
   b. Mobitz II
      (1) S_1 same intensity with stable PR interval
      (2) Pause in rhythm at dropped beat
3. Third-degree A-V block
   a. S_1 with varying intensity, since there is no relationship of PR to QRS
   b. Slow, regular rhythm

In patients with left ventricular dysfunction (myocardial infarction or congestive heart failure), the S_1 is soft. Can you appreciate the changes in intensity of the S_1?

SELF-LEARNING "UNKNOWN" HEART SOUNDS

On the audio program, listen to the "unknown" heart sounds and identify the sound. Compare your answer with the answer key at the end of the chapter. Relisten to the audio program as needed to achieve mastery of the content.

1. Is S$_1$ single or split?

2. Is S$_1$ single or split?

3. Is S$_1$ softer or louder than S$_2$?

4. Is S$_1$ softer or louder than S$_2$?

5. Listen to S$_1$ at the apex with a bell chestpiece and then with a diaphragm chestpiece. Is S$_1$ normal or abnormal?

SELF-LEARNING QUESTIONS

Select the letter of the correct response. Compare your answers with the answer key at the end of the chapter. Reread the chapter as needed to achieve mastery of the content.

1. The S$_1$ results from:
   a. opening of the mitral and tricuspid valves
   b. closing of the mitral and tricuspid valves
   c. opening of the aortic and pulmonic valves
   d. closing of the aortic and pulmonic valves

2. The intensity of S$_1$ would be greater or louder if:
   a. the chest wall were enlarged
   b. less vigor were behind ventricular contraction
   c. the PR interval were short
   d. the mitral valve orifice were open and fixed

3. In a normal split S$_1$, how far apart are the closure sounds?
   a. <0.01 second   b. 0.02 second
   c. 0.04 second   d. >0.04 second

4. The normal split S$_1$ is best heard at:
   a. base right   b. base left
   c. apex   d. LLSB

5. To differentiate S_1 from S_2, which of the following is (are) true?
  (1) At a heart rate of 80 beats/minute or less, S_1 follows the longer pause.
  (2) The S_2 is always loudest at the base.
  (3) With the stethoscope placed on the point of maximal impulse, the sound heard simultaneously with the outward thrust is S_1.
  (4) The sound heard simultaneously with the palpation of the carotid pulse is S_1.
    a. all of the above   **b.** 1 and 3 only
    c. 3 and 4 only   **d.** 2 and 4 only

ANSWERS TO SELF-LEARNING "UNKNOWN" HEART SOUNDS

1. Single S_1

2. Split S_1

3. S_1 louder

4. S_1 softer

5. S_1 normal at apex

ANSWERS TO SELF-LEARNING QUESTIONS

1. b

2. c

3. b

4. d

5. a

3

The Second Heart Sound (S$_2$)

LEARNING OBJECTIVES

After reading this chapter, listening to the accompanying audio program, answering the self-learning questions at the end of the chapter, and listening to the "unknowns" on the audio program, the learner will be able to:

1. Identify the classical theory for the production of the S$_2$.
2. Differentiate between a single S$_2$ and a physiological split S$_2$ (A$_2$P$_2$).
3. Identify the physiology behind the normal physiological splitting of S$_2$.
4. Recognize a normal S$_2$ at the various auscultatory sites.
5. Differentiate between S$_1$ and S$_2$ at the various auscultatory sites.

COMPONENTS OF S_2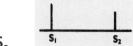

The classical and generally accepted theory for the production of the second heart sound (S_2) is that S_2 is a result of the closure of the aortic (A_2) and pulmonic (P_2) valves. Although some experimental and clinical evidence points to other intracardiac factors contributing to the formation of S_2, the "simple" classical theory is used in this text.

As was true of S_1, the left-sided mechanical event (A_2) has more energy behind its closure and is therefore louder than the right-sided mechanical event (P_2). Also, the left-sided (A_2) normally precedes the right-sided (P_2). The A_2 component is discernible at all the auscultatory sites but is best heard at base right—the site to which aortic sounds radiate best. It is a high-frequency sound and therefore is best heard with the diaphragm applied firmly.

P_2, the second component making up S_2, is the softer of the two components and usually is audible only at base left—the site to which pulmonic sounds radiate best.

PHYSIOLOGICAL SPLIT S_2

If both components that make up S_2 are separately distinguishable, this is known as a *physiological split*. The normal physiological split of S_2 is heard on inspiration; it becomes single on expiration. Thus respiration normally affects the splitting of the S_2 (Figure 3-1). In the physiological split S_2, A_2 and P_2 are about 0.03 second apart. (During inspiration, there is a decrease in intrathoracic pressure that permits an increase in venous return to the right atrium. This increased blood in the right atrium prolongs right ventricular systole and delays pulmonic closing. Because P_2 occurs farther from A_2, the split becomes audible.) The respiratory variation of the physiological split is best appreciated during quiet respiration. If expiration is held, a steady state is rapidly reached until the split of S_2 remains fixed somewhere between the width on inspiration and expiration.

As people age, the degree of normal inspiratory splitting of S_2 decreases, so many older people do not demonstrate audible inspiratory splitting of S_2. The absence of an audible split on inspiration does not indicate a pathology, but a distinctly audible splitting of S_2 on expiration is abnormal.

Listen now to a physiological split S_2—split audible on inspiration; sound single on expiration. A split S_2 is normal, or physiological, only if the split occurs during inspiration and becomes single during

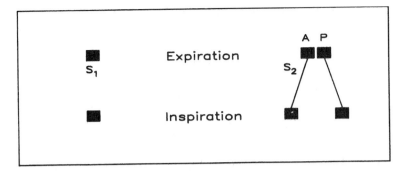

Figure 3-1   Physiological splitting of the second heart sound *(S₂)*. (Reproduced with permission from Caccamo L, Erickson B: *Cardiac auscultation*, Youngstown, Ohio, 1975, St. Elizabeth's Hospital Medical Center.)

expiration. It is normal also if the split is not audible. Listen again to an S₂ that is split and an S₂ that is single (only aortic component audible).

S₂ AUSCULTATORY VARIATIONS

 Listen now to the normal S₂ at the various auscultatory sites:
1. LLSB—single S₂
2. Apex—single S₂
3. Base right—single S₂
4. Base left—split S₂ on inspiration; single S₂ on expiration

The loudness, or intensity, of S₂ also changes, depending on the site auscultated. S₂ is always loudest at base right or base left. It is softer than S₁ at the LLSB and the apex.

INTENSITY OF S₂

 Listen to the loudness of the normal S₂ at the various auscultatory sites:
1. LLSB—S₂ softer than S₁
2. Apex—S₂ softer than S₁
3. Base right—S₂ louder than S₁
4. Base left—S₂ louder than S₁

When listening to the normal S₂, the following occurs at each specified site:
1. LLSB—single S₂; S₂ softer than S₁
2. Apex—single S₂; S₂ softer than S₁

3. Base right—single S_2; S_2 louder than S_1
4. Base left—split S_2 on inspiration (A_2P_2); single S_2 on expiration (or always single); S_2 louder than S_1

NORMAL S_1 AND S_2

 Review now the normal S_1 and S_2 for each specified site:

	S_1	S_2
LLSB	Single or split; louder	Single; softer
Apex	Single; louder	Single; softer
Base right	Single; softer	Single; louder
Base left	Single; softer	Split on inspiration; single on expiration; louder

CLINICAL CORRELATION

When you are confident in your ability to discern S_2, practice it in the clinical area. As you did with S_1, listen to as many different individuals as possible (e.g., children, adults, thin, obese). Pay special attention to S_2. Can you identify whether S_2 is single or physiologically split? Note the difference in intensity, depending on the site auscultated. Can you differentiate S_2 from S_1? Listen selectively to S_2, but listen also to S_1. Practice recording both S_1 and S_2 on an auscultogram.

Practice hearing the normal physiological split S_2 that splits on inspiration and is single on expiration. You will hear it at base left. If you do not hear the split, do not think that something is wrong. The physiological split is not audible in everyone, but to be normal the split must occur on inspiration.

SELF-LEARNING "UNKNOWN" HEART SOUNDS

 On the audio program, listen to the "unknown" heart sounds and identify the sound. Compare your answer with the answer key at the end of the chapter. Relisten to the audio program as needed to achieve mastery of the content.

1. Is S_2 single or physiologically split?

2. Is S_2 single or physiologically split?

3. Is S_1 or S_2 split?

4. Is S_1 or S_2 split?

5. Listen to S_2 at base right with a bell chestpiece and then with a diaphragm chestpiece. Is S_2 normal or abnormal?

SELF-LEARNING QUESTIONS

Select the letter of the correct response. Compare your answers with the answer key at the end of the chapter. Reread the chapter as needed to achieve mastery of the content.

1. The normal S_2 is produced by:
   a. opening of aortic and pulmonic valves
   b. closing of aortic and pulmonic valves
   c. opening of mitral and tricuspid valves
   d. closing of mitral and tricuspid valves

2. The physiological splitting of S_2 relates to the fact that during inspiration:
   a. closure of pulmonic valve is delayed
   b. opening of pulmonic valve is delayed
   c. closure of aortic valve is delayed
   d. opening of aortic valve is delayed

3. In the normal heart, when listening at base right, S_1 is single; S_2 is:
   a. split and softer than S_1
   b. split and louder than S_1
   c. single and softer than S_1
   d. single and louder than S_1

4. In the normal heart, when listening at base left, the physiological splitting of S_2 occurs during:
   a. inspiration
   b. expiration
   c. both inspiration and expiration
   d. none of the above

5. In the normal heart, S_2 is louder than S_1 at:
   a. LLSB
   b. apex
   c. base right or left
   d. base left only

ANSWERS TO SELF-LEARNING "UNKNOWN" HEART SOUNDS

1. Single S_2

2. Physiologically split S_2

3. Split S_1

4. Split S_2

5. Normal S_2 at base right

ANSWERS TO SELF-LEARNING QUESTIONS

1. b

2. a

3. d

4. a

5. c

4

The Fourth Heart Sound (S$_4$)

LEARNING OBJECTIVES

After reading this chapter, listening to the accompanying audio program, answering the self-learning questions at the end of the chapter, and listening to the "unknowns" on the audio program, the learner will be able to:

1. Identify the characteristics of S$_4$.
2. Identify the physiology behind the production of S$_4$.
3. Choose the correct chestpiece of the stethoscope for listening to S$_4$.
4. Differentiate right ventricular S$_4$ from left ventricular S$_4$.
5. Differentiate a normal split S$_1$ from an S$_4$.

NOMENCLATURE OF S$_4$

The diastolic sound heard just before S$_1$ is known by the following terms: *fourth heart sound, atrial gallop, presystolic gallop, S$_4$ gallop,* and *S$_4$*. The term *gallop* is used because at a rapid heart rate the presence of the S$_4$ in the cardiac sequence resembles the canter of a horse. *Atrial gallop* is a misleading term, since the implication is that the atrium is the source of the extra sound when in fact the sound comes from the ventricle(s). S$_4$ is the most commonly used term.

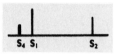

COMPONENTS OF S$_4$

S$_4$ is a low-frequency sound heard just before S$_1$. Because it is a sound of low frequency, it is best heard with the bell held lightly. S$_4$ is a result of decreased ventricular compliance or increased volume of filling. It is a sign of ventricular stress.

S$_4$ is a diastolic sound that occurs during the late diastolic filling phase (the time at which "atrial kick" occurs). Ventricles receiving this additional blood from the atrium may generate a low-frequency vibration—the S$_4$. This occurs if the ventricles have a decreased compliance or are receiving an increased diastolic volume. An S$_4$ does not occur unless atrial contraction takes place. Therefore an S$_4$ is never heard in atrial fibrillation.

S$_4$ normally may be heard in an athletic person younger than 20 years because of the increased diastolic volume that is normal in the young. S$_4$ also may be indicative of an abnormality of the heart (myocardial infarction is associated with decreased ventricular compliance).

S$_4$ may be of either left or right ventricular origin. S$_4$ of left ventricular origin is best heard at the apex during expiration, with the patient in the supine or left lateral recumbent position. (Sounds from the left part of the heart radiate best to the apex. Having the patient supine increases the volume of blood in the ventricles, making S$_4$ louder. Turning the patient to the left lateral recumbent position brings the heart closer to the chest, also making S$_4$ louder.) Common causes of an S$_4$ of left ventricular origin are severe hypertension, aortic stenosis, primary myocardial disease, coronary artery disease, and cardiomyopathy. S$_4$ is heard also in conditions with increased cardiac output and stroke volume, such as thyrotoxicosis or anemia.

S$_4$ of right ventricular origin is best heard at the left lateral sternal border (LLSB) and is accentuated with inspiration. (Sounds from the right part of the heart radiate best to the LLSB. During inspiration, an increased volume of blood is returned to the right atrium and the right ventricle, making S$_4$ louder.) S$_4$ may reflect pulmonary valve obstruction, pulmonary stenosis, or pulmonic hypertension.

Dysrhythmias also may affect the presence or absence of S_4. S_4 may be heard when the PR interval is prolonged (0.22 second or longer) and commonly is heard in first-, second-, or third-degree atrial-ventricular (A-V) block. With the prolonged PR interval, S_4 is not buried in the first sound or heard in conjunction with it. S_4 is never heard in atrial fibrillation, since atrial contraction does not occur in this dysrhythmia.

S_4 is audible with the bell held lightly. (Pressure on the bell causes the skin to be stretched tightly across the bottom of the bell, turning it into a diaphragm.) Thus firm pressure on the bell will cause S_4 to diminish or to disappear.

 Listen now to an S_4. Initially only S_1 and S_2 will be heard, and then S_4 will be added. Listen to S_4 with the bell held lightly and then to S_4 with the bell applied firmly (note that S_4 disappears).

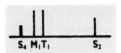

DIFFERENTIATING S₄ FROM SPLIT S₁

 S_4:

    1. Low frequency before S_1
    2. Best heard with bell held lightly
    3. Pressure on bell causes S_4 to diminish or disappear
Split S_1 (M_1T_1) has the following characteristics:
    1. High frequency
    2. Best heard with diaphragm or bell applied firmly
    3. Sounds 0.02 second apart

S_4 can be decreased by reducing the blood return to the atrium (by standing). S_4 can be increased by increasing atrial blood return (by coughing, squatting, or elevating the legs) or by bringing the heart closer to the stethoscope (by rolling the patient to the left lateral recumbent position). If S_4 occurs from the right ventricle, it may become louder with inspiration.

A split S_1 may be increased on standing but is not significantly affected by the other maneuvers.

 Again listen to an S_4 compared to a split S_1. Listen to a single S_1; then S_1 split; then an S_4 in front of the split S_1. Then listen to a split S_1 with an S_4 taken in and out.

CLINICAL CORRELATION

Clinical practice in listening to S_4 can be obtained by selecting patients with conditions most likely to have an S_4. Patients with primary myocardial disease, coronary artery disease, cardiomyopathy, aortic stenosis, or severe hypertension may have an S_4 of left ventricular origin that is best heard at the apex. An S_4 of right ventricular origin may be heard in a patient with pulmonary valve obstruction, pulmonary stenosis, or pulmonic hypertension. This S_4 is best heard at the LLSB. Coronary care units are an ideal place to hear an S_4. (Remember that patients with atrial fibrillation can not have S_4.) S_4 changes its intensity and distance from S_1 during the various stages of myocardial infarction: (1) initially the S_4 is loud and occurs farther from S_1; (2) as healing occurs and ventricular compliance improves, S_4 becomes softer and closer to S_1 (therefore harder to hear); (3) if the patient has a reinfarction or an extension, S_4 again is loud and occurs farther from S_1. Therefore, in the progression of an uncomplicated myocardial infarction, you would expect S_4 initially to be easy to hear and gradually to become less and less perceptible. Also listen to athletic children who may have an S_4 that is normal. The auscultatory findings between the "normal" S_4 in children and the "pathological" S_4 are similar. The clinical history differentiates the normal S_4 from the pathological S_4. Do not be discouraged if you have difficulty hearing an S_4 in the clinical area. The S_4 is one of the most difficult sounds to hear, since it is just within the acoustical ability of the ear. To bring out S_4, have the patient do a mild exercise such as coughing or turning to the left side. Turning to the left lateral recumbent position also brings the heart closer to the chest wall and makes S_4 easier to hear. Also listen to S_1 and S_2. Practice recording S_1, S_2, and S_4 on an auscultogram.

SELF-LEARNING "UNKNOWN" HEART SOUNDS

 On the audio program, listen to the "unknown" heart sounds and identify the sound. Compare your answer with the answer key at the end of the chapter. Relisten to the audio program as needed to achieve mastery of the content.

You are listening to the heart at the LLSB:
    Using the bell held lightly, what do you hear?
    Using the bell applied firmly, what do you hear?
    Using the diaphragm, what do you hear?

  1. Is S_1 single or split?
    Is there an S_4?

You are listening to the heart at the LLSB:
    Using the bell held lightly, what do you hear?

Using the bell applied firmly, what do you hear?
Using the diaphragm, what do you hear?

2. Is the S_1 single or split?
   Is there an S_4?

You are listening to the heart at the apex:
   Using the bell held lightly, what do you hear?
   Using the bell applied firmly, what do you hear?
   Using the diaphragm, what do you hear?

3. Is S_1 single or split?
   Is there an S_4?

You are listening to the heart at the apex:
   Using the bell held lightly, what do you hear?
   Using the bell applied firmly, what do you hear?
   Using the diaphragm, what do you hear?

4. Is the S_1 single or split?
   Is there an S_4?

You are listening to the heart at the LLSB:
   Using the bell held lightly, what do you hear?
   Using the bell applied firmly, what do you hear?
   Using the diaphragm, what do you hear?

5. When listening with the bell held lightly:
   Is the S_1 single or split?
   Is there an S_4?

SELF-LEARNING QUESTIONS

Select the letter of the correct response. Compare your answers with the answer key at the end of the chapter. Reread the chapter as needed to achieve mastery of the content.

1. The S_4 is of
   a. low frequency
   b. high frequency
   c. medium frequency
   d. rough frequency

2. S_4 occurs during which phase of the cardiac cycle?
   a. early systolic filling   b. late systolic filling
   c. early diastolic filling   d. late diastolic filling

3. You are listening to a patient with atrial fibrillation. You know that an S_4 in this patient is
   a. louder than normal   b. softer than normal
   c. always heard   d. never heard

4. Which of the following options would you choose to hear an S_4 best?
   a. bell firmly pressed   b. bell lightly held
   c. diaphragm firmly pressed   d. diaphragm lightly held

5. An S_4 of left ventricular origin would be best heard at
   a. base right   b. base left
   c. apex   d. LLSB

ANSWERS TO SELF-LEARNING "UNKNOWN" HEART SOUNDS

1. Split S_1; no S_4

2. Single S_1; with S_4

3. Single S_1; no S_4

4. Single S_1; with S_4

5. Split S_1; with S_4

ANSWERS TO SELF-LEARNING QUESTIONS

1. a

2. d

3. d

4. b

5. c

C·H·A·P·T·E·R

5

The Third Heart Sound (S$_3$)

LEARNING OBJECTIVES

After reading this chapter, listening to the accompanying audio program, answering the self-learning questions at the end of the chapter, and listening to the "unknowns" on the audio program, the learner will be able to:

1. Identify the characteristics of S$_3$.
2. Identify the physiology behind the production of S$_3$.
3. Choose the correct chestpiece of the stethoscope for listening to S$_3$.
4. Differentiate a right ventricular S$_3$ from a left ventricular S$_3$.
5. Differentiate a physiological split S$_2$ (A$_2$P$_2$) from S$_3$.
6. Differentiate S$_3$ from S$_4$.

NOMENCLATURE OF S₃

The third heart sound has been known as *ventricular gallop, protodiastolic gallop, S₃ gallop,* and *S₃.* The term *gallop* was used because the sequence of heart sounds with an S₃ or S₄ resembles the canter of a horse, especially when the heart is beating rapidly.

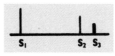

COMPONENTS OF S₃

S₃ is a low-frequency sound heard just after the S₂. Because it is of low frequency, it is best heard with the bell held lightly. S₃ is a result of decreased ventricular compliance or increased ventricular diastolic volume. It may be a sign of ventricular distress, or trouble, as in congestive heart failure. S₃ is a diastolic sound that occurs during the early rapid filling phase of ventricular filling.

S₃ is normal in children and young adults because they have increased diastolic volumes. Men tend to lose S₃ in their 20s; women lose S₃ in their 30s. An S₃ after the age of 40 usually is associated with cardiac disease except in those individuals physically active in sports. It is heard also in patients with coronary artery disease, cardiomyopathy, incompetent valves, and left-to-right shunts (ventricular septal defect or patent ductus arteriosus) and is the first clinical sign of congestive heart failure. The preceding conditions may cause a decrease in ventricular compliance, an increase in left ventricular diastolic volume, or both.

S₃ may have its origin in either the right or left ventricle—the latter being more common. Left S₃ is best heard at the apex. (Sounds from the left side of the heart are best heard at the apex because this is the area to which they radiate.)

Right S₃ is best heard at the left lateral sternal border (LLSB) or xiphoid area. (Sounds from the right heart are best heard at the LLSB or xiphoid because this is the area to which they radiate.)

 Listen now to S₃. Initially only S₁ and S₂ will be heard, and then S₃ will be added.

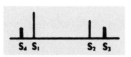

DIFFERENTIATING S₃ FROM S₄

 Timing permits S₃ to be distinguished from S₄:
1. S₃ comes after S₂
2. S₄ comes before S₁

In some individuals, both S_3 and S_4 may be present. If the heart rate is normal (60 to 100 beats/min) and both S_3 and S_4 are present, a **quadruple rhythm** can be heard (four-sound cadence). At a rapid rate, S_3 and S_4 may occur simultaneously and are heard as a very loud diastolic sound known as a **summation gallop**. This fusion of S_3 and S_4 occurs because the tachycardia shortens diastole.

For a synopsis of the various sounds that can occur around S_2 and a method of differentiating one from the other, see Table 10-1.

CLINICAL CORRELATION

Clinical practice in listening to S_3 can be obtained by selecting patients with conditions most likely to have an S_3. As was true of S_4, the coronary care unit is one of the best places to hear the pathological S_3. Remember that S_3 is the first clinical sign of congestive heart failure. S_3 is normal in children and young adults. The auscultatory findings between the "normal" S_3 and the "pathological" S_3 are similar. The clinical history differentiates the normal S_3 from the pathological S_3. S_3 is easier to hear than S_4, but you still may need to make S_3 more perceptible by having the patient do a mild exercise such as coughing or turning to the left side. Changing the patient's position from sitting to supine also may bring out S_3. (This is true also of S_4.) Having the patient grip one hand with the other also may bring out S_3 (or S_4). The handgrip increases peripheral vascular resistance, blood pressure, heart rate, and cardiac output. Also listen to S_1, S_2, and S_4. Can you differentiate the split S_1 from an S_4; the physiological split S_2 from S_3; S_4 from S_3? Practice recording the S_1, S_2, S_3, and S_4 on an auscultogram.

SELF-LEARNING "UNKNOWN" HEART SOUNDS

 On the audio program, listen to the "unknown" heart sounds and identify the sound. Compare your answer with the answer key at the end of the chapter. Relisten to the audio program as needed to achieve mastery of the content.

You are listening to the heart at the apex:
Using the bell held lightly, what do you hear?
Using the bell applied firmly, what do you hear?
Using the diaphragm, what do you hear?

1. Is S_2 single, split, or is there an S_3?

You are listening to the heart at base left:
    Using the bell held lightly, what do you hear?
    Using the bell applied firmly, what do you hear?
    Using the diaphragm, what do you hear?

2. Is S_2 single, split, or is there an S_3?

You are listening to the heart at the apex:
    Using the bell held lightly, what do you hear?
    Using the bell applied firmly, what do you hear?
    Using the diaphragm, what do you hear?

3. Is there an S_4 or S_3?

You are listening to the heart at the apex:
    Using the bell held lightly, what do you hear?
    Using the bell applied firmly, what do you hear?
    Using the diaphragm, what do you hear?

4. Is there an S_4 or S_3?

You are listening to the heart at the apex:
    Using the bell held lightly, what do you hear?
    Using the bell applied firmly, what do you hear?
    Using the diaphragm, what do you hear?

5. Is there an S_4 or S_3?

SELF-LEARNING QUESTIONS

Select the letter of the correct response. Compare your answers with the answer key at the end of the chapter. Reread the chapter as needed to achieve mastery of the content.

1. S_3 is a low-frequency sound that is best heard with which chestpiece of the stethoscope?
    a. bell held lightly   b. bell applied firmly
    c. diaphragm held lightly   d. diaphragm applied firmly

2. S_3 is the result of _____ ventricular compliance or _____ ventricular diastolic volume.
    a. increased; increased   b. decreased; increased
    c. increased; decreased   d. decreased; decreased

3. S_3 is heard in an 8-year-old boy with no other abnormal clinical findings. You consider the third heart sound to be:

   a. abnormal, needing consultation

   b. abnormal, watch closely

   c. never normal

   d. normal in children

4. S_3 of left ventricular origin would be best heard at:

   a. base right

   b. base left

   c. apex

   d. left lateral sternal border

5. The first clinical sign of congestive heart failure is:

   a. S_4

   b. wide split S_1

   c. S_3

   d. wide split S_2

ANSWERS TO SELF-LEARNING "UNKNOWN" HEART SOUNDS

1. Single S_2 with S_3

2. Physiological split S_2

3. S_4

4. S_3

5. S_4 and S_3

ANSWERS TO SELF-LEARNING QUESTIONS

1. a

2. b

3. d

4. c

5. c

6

Murmurs—General Information

LEARNING OBJECTIVES

After reading this chapter, listening to the accompanying audio program, answering the self-learning questions at the end of the chapter, and listening to the "unknowns" on the audio program, the learner will be able to:

1. Define a murmur.
2. Identify the common causes of murmurs.
3. Identify the six characteristics to be considered in murmur identification.
4. Classify murmurs using a one-through-six classification scale.
5. Differentiate between murmurs of high, medium, and low frequency.
6. Differentiate between murmurs having the quality of "blowing," "harsh," "rough," or "rumble."
7. Differentiate between systolic and diastolic murmurs.

CHARACTERISTICS OF MURMURS

Murmurs are defined as sustained noises that are audible during the time periods of systole, diastole, or both.

Common causes of murmurs include backward regurgitation (a leaking valve, atrial or ventricular septal defect, or arteriovenous connection); forward flow through narrowed or deformed valves; a high rate of blood flow through normal or abnormal valves; vibration of loose structures within the heart (chordae tendineae); and continuous flow through atrial-ventricular (A-V) shunts.

To identify a murmur, you need to consider six characteristics:
1. Location—valve area where murmur best heard
2. Loudness (intensity)—use the one-through-six grading system
3. Frequency (pitch)—i.e., low, medium, high
4. Quality—blowing, harsh or rough, or rumble
5. Timing—systolic or diastolic
6. Radiation—where else murmur heard

CLASSIFICATION OF MURMURS

Murmurs are usually classified using a I-through-VI (one-through-six) grading scale and recorded with the grade heard over the scale used (i.e., I/VI or 1/6):

I/VI Sound not audible first few seconds (listener must tune in before hearing)

II/VI Sound heard at once but faint

III/VI Sound loud but without thrust or thrill*

IV/VI Sound loud with thrust or thrill

V/VI Sound loud with thrust or thrill and audible with chestpiece tilted or partly off chest

VI/VI Sound loud with thrust or thrill and audible with chestpiece off chest

LOCATION OF MURMURS

The location of murmurs, as with normal heart sounds, originates near a heart valve. You will find it necessary to listen to the four basic areas previously discussed, plus a fifth area, commonly called *Erb's point*, which

---

Thrust when clinician palpates precordium the sensation taps hand and falls away. *Thrill* when clinician palpates precordium and sensation is similar to placing hand on a purring cat.

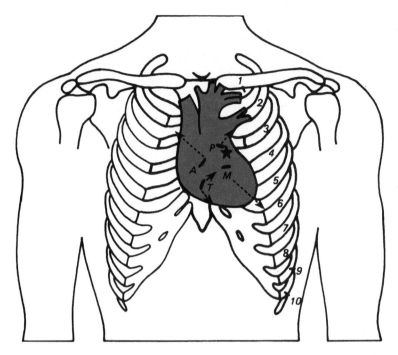

Figure 6-1   Valve areas. *Anatomic* area is represented by *solid bars.* M, Mitral valve; *T,* tricuspid valve; *A,* aortic valve; *P,* pulmonic valve. *Auscultatory* areas (areas where sound is heard best) are represented by *arrows. Star* (★) represents Erb's point.

is located at the third intercostal space (3 ICS) along the left lateral sternal border (LLSB) (Figure 6-1).

To determine murmur location, listen to all the basic areas and decide at which area the murmur is best heard. You will find that murmurs from certain valves tend to be best heard "downstream" from the valve:

Valve	Best Heard
1. Mitral	Apex
2. Tricuspid	LLSB
3. Pulmonic	Base left
4. Aortic (systolic)	Base right
Aortic (diastolic)	Erb's point

LOUDNESS OF MURMURS

Loudness (intensity) is judged by using the same one-through-six classification previously discussed for heart sounds. The loudness of the murmur should not be thought to correlate with its significance. Some insignificant abnormalities may have loud murmurs, whereas the same

TABLE 6-1
Differentiation of Common Cardiac Abnormalities by Pitch and Quality

Pitch	Frequency (cycles/sec)	Quality	Abnormality	Chestpiece
High	200-400	Blowing	Mitral regurgitation Tricuspid regurgitation Aortic regurgitation Ventricular septal defect (VSD)	Diaphragm
Medium	100-200	Harsh Rough	Aortic stenosis Pulmonic regurgitation Atrial Septal defect (ASD) Increase flow of pulmonary outflow tract	Either Bell
Low	<100	Rumble	Mitral stenosis	Bell

Modified with permission from Caccamo L, Erickson B: *Cardiac auscultation*, Youngstown, Ohio 1975, St. Elizabeth's Hospital Medical Center.

abnormality that has progressed in significance may be softer. (Think of a plaque occluding an artery. Minimal plaque may have intense sustained noise [bruit]; complete occlusion may have no sound.)

FREQUENCY OF MURMURS

Frequency (pitch) indicates whether the sound heard is high, medium, or low. This is easily determined, since (1) murmurs of high frequency are best heard with the diaphragm chestpiece, (2) those of low frequency are best heard with the bell held lightly, and (3) those of medium frequency are best heard with either bell or diaphragm chestpiece. With practice, the frequency of the murmur will alert you to the presence of a specific abnormality (Table 6-1).

 Listen now to murmurs that are considered high, medium, and low.

QUALITY OF MURMURS

Quality is closely related to frequency and is described as "blowing" (mainly high frequency); "harsh" or "rough" (medium frequency—mix of high and low frequencies); and "rumble" (mainly low frequency). The quality of the murmur alerts the astute clinician to the presence of a specific abnormality (see Table 6-1).

 Listen now to murmurs that are described as "blowing," "harsh" or "rough," and "rumble." For a differentiation of the common murmurs by frequency and quality, see Table 6-1.

TIMING OF MURMURS

Timing means that you can identify whether the sustained noise is occurring between S_1 and S_2—a systolic murmur; or between S_2 and S_1—a diastolic murmur. In some abnormalities the murmur will be heard in both systole and diastole.

 Listen now to a heart rate of 60 beats/minute. First, a systolic blow murmur will be added and then removed. Then a diastolic rumble murmur will be added and removed. Murmurs of different frequency and quality have been deliberately selected to help you tell the difference between systole and diastole.

As a beginning auscultator, you may not be able to pinpoint the timing any more precisely than to determine whether the murmur occurs in systole or diastole. However, with experience you will note that even "finer timing" (early, mid, late, or pan) is possible. A murmur is said to be *early* if its peak intensity occurs early in the cycle; *mid* if the peak intensity occurs in the middle of the cycle; and *late* if the peak intensity occurs late in the cycle. If the murmur is heard throughout the cycle with equal intensity, it is known as a *pan* or *holo* murmur.

 Listen now to a heart rate of 60 beats/minute. A murmur will be added in the systolic period: early, mid, late, and pan.

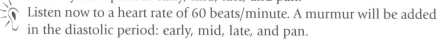 Listen now to a heart rate of 60 beats/minute. A murmur will be added in the diastolic period: early, mid, late, and pan.

RADIATION OF MURMURS

Radiation of the murmur is assessed when you determine in what other areas the sound is audible in addition to where you heard it best. Each cardiac abnormality has a classical radiation. See Figures 7-1 and 8-1 for the radiation patterns of common cardiac abnormalities.

SHAPE OF MURMURS

Murmurs have an identifiable shape to their sound that is often described in musical terminology. A *crescendo/decrescendo* (diamond-shaped) murmur starts softly, peaks in intensity, and then diminishes (systolic murmur of aortic stenosis). A *decrescendo* murmur begins loud and gets progressively quieter (diastolic murmur of aortic regurgitation). A *pan* or *holo* murmur remains unchanged from the onset to the end of the sound (pansystolic murmur of severe mitral regurgitation). A *crescendo* murmur starts out soft and becomes progressively louder (late systolic murmur of mitral valve prolapse). A *decrescendo/crescendo* murmur starts out loud, gets softer, and then becomes loud again (diastolic murmur of mitral stenosis).

SPECIAL MANEUVERS

Special maneuvers to help differentiate one murmur (or sound) from another include Valsalva, exercise, respiration, handgrip, and the use of amyl nitrate. The **Valsalva** is performed by asking the patient to bear down or strain. This maneuver increases intrathoracic pressure and decreases venous return to the right heart. Most murmurs decrease during the strain phase of the Valsalva. After release of the straining phase, right-sided events return in 1 to 3 beats, whereas left-sided events return in 4 to 11 beats. **Exercise** increases the heart rate and thereby increases blood flow; murmurs (and sounds) may be increased in intensity. Respiration also changes the loudness of sounds by bringing the heart closer to the chest wall and making the heart sounds louder. Therefore faint diastolic murmurs of aortic or pulmonic regurgitation may be heard better during expiration.* **Handgrip** in which one hand is gripped with the other causes an increase in peripheral vascular resistance, blood pressure, heart rate, and cardiac output. This maneuver increases left-sided regurgitant murmurs (aortic and mitral regurgitation and ventricular septal defect) and decreases left-sided ejection murmurs (aortic stenosis). **Amyl nitrate** decreases peripheral vascular resistance and increases heart rate and venous return. After inhalation of amyl nitrate, forward flow murmurs (aortic stenosis, mitral stenosis, pulmonic stenosis, and tricuspid stenosis) increase; left-sided regurgitant murmurs become softer.

---

*This is not to be confused with the physiological effects of respiration. During inspiration right-sided cardiac events are louder because of the increased venous return.

SELF-LEARNING "UNKNOWN" HEART SOUNDS

 On the audio program, listen to the "unknown" heart sounds and identify the sound. Compare your answer with the answer key at the end of the chapter. Relisten to the audio program as needed to achieve mastery of the content.

Determine the frequency of the following sustained sounds.

1. This sound is best heard with the diaphragm applied firmly.

2. This sound is heard equally well with either the bell or the diaphragm.

3. This sound is best heard with the bell held lightly. Determine the quality of the following sounds.

4. This sound is best heard with the diaphragm applied firmly.

5. This sound is best heard with the bell held lightly.

SELF-LEARNING QUESTIONS

Select the letter of the correct response, or provide requested information. Compare your answers with the answer key at the end of the chapter. Reread the chapter as needed to achieve mastery of the content.

1. A sustained noise that is audible during the time period of systole, diastole, or both periods is descriptive of:
   a. systolic murmur   **b.** diastolic murmur
   c. murmur   **d.** blow

2. Name two common causes for murmur production.
   a.
   b.

3. Name the six characteristics you need to consider to identify a murmur.
   a.
   b.
   c.
   d.
   e.
   f.

4. If the sustained noise occurs between S_1 and S_2, the murmur is called:
   a. systolic   b. diastolic
   c. regurgitant   d. ejection

ANSWERS TO SELF-LEARNING "UNKNOWN" HEART SOUNDS

1. High frequency

2. Medium frequency

3. Low frequency

4. Blowing

5. Rumble

ANSWERS TO SELF-LEARNING QUESTIONS

1. c

2. Any two:
   —Backward regurgitation
   —Forward flow through narrow or deformed valves
   —High rate of blood flow through normal or abnormal valves
   —Vibration of loose structures within the heart

3. —Location
   —Loudness
   —Frequency
   —Quality
   —Timing
   —Radiation

4. a

7

Systolic Murmurs

LEARNING OBJECTIVES

After reading this chapter, listening to the accompanying audio program, answering the self-learning questions at the end of the chapter, and listening to the "unknowns" on the audio program, the learner will be able to:

1. Define systolic murmur.
2. Identify the mechanism(s) of systolic murmur production.
3. Identify the characteristics of an early systolic, midsystolic, late systolic, and pansystolic murmur.
4. Differentiate between an early systolic, midsystolic, late systolic, and pansystolic murmur.
5. Identify common adult abnormalities having systolic murmurs.

Systolic murmurs are sustained noises that are audible between S_1 and S_2. In some patients, systolic murmurs may be normal. This may be true of infants or children because of their thin chest walls. In adults, a "normal" systolic murmur may be the result of increased blood flow, as in pregnancy. A systolic murmur probably would be heard in most normal hearts if listened for in a soundproof room.

MECHANISM(S) OF SYSTOLIC MURMUR PRODUCTION

Systolic murmurs occur during the ventricular systolic period. Forward flow across the aortic or pulmonic valve or regurgitant flow from the mitral or tricuspid valve may produce a systolic murmur. The valves may be normal (but with a high rate of flow) or abnormal. Common abnormalities in which a systolic murmur is heard include mitral insufficiency, tricuspid insufficiency, aortic stenosis, pulmonic stenosis, and interventricular septal defects.

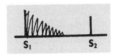

EARLY SYSTOLIC MURMURS

An early systolic murmur begins with S_1 and peaks in the first third of systole. It may be caused by a modified regurgitant murmur with backward flow through an incompetent valve, a septal defect, or an atrial-ventricular (A-V) communication. Common causes are a small ventricular septal defect or the "innocent" murmurs of children.

Listen now to a heart rate of 60 beats/minute. Then an early systolic murmur will be added.

An **innocent** systolic murmur usually is either early or ejection (see Midsystolic Murmurs). Its grade is a 2/6 or less. It is common in children. This sound is considered normal or "innocent" if there is no recognizable heart lesion and if:
1. Normal split S_2 is heard (S_2 splits on inspiration; single on expiration).
2. Normal jugular venous and carotid pulses are present.
3. Normal precordial pulsation is present.
4. History, chest x-ray, and electrocardiogram (ECG) are normal.

Common causes are:
1. Pulmonary outflow tract murmur (ejection)
2. Vibratory (humming or musical) that is heard in children (ages 2 to 7 years) at the left lateral sternal border (LLSB)

Innocent systolic murmurs may be heard also in the elderly—most commonly a result of sclerotic changes of the aortic valve. The murmur usually is of short duration and faint, with a grade of 2/6 or less. The "innocent" murmur of the elderly may continue a benign course for years or gradually progress and cause symptoms. Other causes of innocent systolic murmurs include conditions in which blood flow is increased, such as hyperthyroidism, anemia, fever, exercise, and pregnancy (92%).

 Listen now to a heart rate of 60 beats/minute. An early innocent murmur will be added. The early systolic murmur will be compared with a midsystolic murmur.

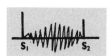

MIDSYSTOLIC MURMURS

A midsystolic murmur begins shortly after S_1, peaks in midsystole, and does not quite extend to S_2. It is known as an *ejection* murmur. It is a *crescendo/decrescendo* murmur (diamond-shaped) that builds up and decreases symmetrically. It may be caused by forward blood flow through a narrow or irregular valve such as that found in aortic or pulmonic stenosis.

 Listen now to a heart rate of 60 beats/minute. A midsystolic murmur will be added, which is medium in frequency and harsh in quality.

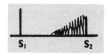

LATE SYSTOLIC MURMURS

A late systolic murmur begins in the latter half of systole, peaks in the later third of systole, and extends to S_2. It is a modified regurgitant murmur with a backward flow through an incompetent valve. It commonly is heard in papillary muscle disorders and in the mitral valve prolapse syndrome.

 Listen now to a heart rate of 60 beats/minute. A late systolic murmur will be added that is high in frequency and blowing in quality.

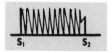

PANSYSTOLIC (OR HOLOSYSTOLIC) MURMURS

A pansystolic (or holosystolic) murmur is heard continuously throughout systole. It begins with S_1 and ends with S_2. Because the pressure remains higher throughout systole in the ejecting chamber than in the receiving chamber, the murmur is continuous. It is commonly heard in mitral regurgitation, tricuspid regurgitation, and ventricular septal defect.

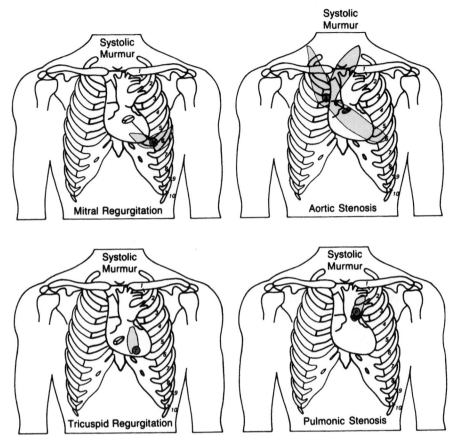

Figure 7-1   Common cardiac abnormalities with systolic murmur(s). Area where murmur is heard best is *circled*; area of usual radiation is *shaded*.

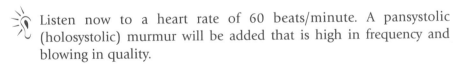 Listen now to a heart rate of 60 beats/minute. A pansystolic (holosystolic) murmur will be added that is high in frequency and blowing in quality.

A review of the common adult abnormalities having systolic murmurs is provided in Figure 7-1.

CLINICAL CORRELATION

One of the easiest ways to gain clinical practice in listening to systolic murmurs is to seek out patients in whom these murmurs already have been identified. Common pathologies having this type of murmur are mitral regurgitation, tricuspid regurgitation, aortic stenosis, and pulmonic stenosis. Patients with mitral valve prolapse may have a late systolic murmur. Systolic murmurs also may be heard in normal hearts. Initially, try to determine whether the murmur is in systole or in diastole. With practice you will be able to tell whether it is in early systole, midsystole, or late systole. Also determine the following: (1) location—valve area where best heard; (2) loudness; (3) frequency; (4) quality; and (5) radiation. Practice recording the systolic murmur on an auscultogram. Also practice writing a narrative description of the systolic murmur heard.

Keep in mind that murmurs originating on the right side of the heart generally increase with inspiration and that those from the left side decrease. You also may wish to try some of the maneuvers described in Special Maneuvers in Chapter 6.

Chapter 12, Prosthetic Valve Sounds, contains information about how a systolic ejection murmur can be heard with prosthetic valves.

SELF-LEARNING "UNKNOWN" HEART SOUNDS

 On the audio program, listen to the "unknown" heart sounds and identify the sound. Compare your answers with the answer key at the end of the chapter. Relisten to the audio program as needed to achieve mastery of the content.

Listen to the following systolic murmurs.

1. Is the murmur early systolic, midsystolic, late systolic, or pansystolic in nature?

2. Is the murmur early systolic, midsystolic, late systolic, or pansystolic in nature?

3. Is the murmur early systolic, midsystolic, late systolic, or pansystolic in nature?

4. Is the murmur early systolic, midsystolic, late systolic, or pansystolic in nature?

5. Is the quality of this late systolic murmur blowing or rumble?

SELF-LEARNING QUESTIONS

Select the letter of the correct response. Compare your answers with the answer key at the end of the chapter. Reread the chapter as needed to achieve mastery of the content.

1. Sustained noises that are audible between the S_1 and S_2 are descriptive of:
   - **a.** systolic murmur
   - **c.** ejection sound
   - **b.** diastolic murmur
   - **d.** friction rub

2. Regurgitant blood flow across which valves will cause a systolic murmur?
   - **a.** mitral and aortic
   - **c.** tricuspid and pulmonic
   - **b.** mitral and tricuspid
   - **d.** pulmonic and aortic

3. Forward blood flow across which abnormal valves will cause a systolic murmur?
   - **a.** mitral and aortic
   - **c.** tricuspid and pulmonic
   - **b.** mitral and tricuspid
   - **d.** pulmonic and aortic

4. Common adult abnormalities having a systolic murmur include:
   - **a.** mitral insufficiency and aortic insufficiency
   - **b.** mitral stenosis and aortic insufficiency
   - **c.** mitral insufficiency and aortic stenosis
   - **d.** mitral stenosis and aortic stenosis

5. A murmur that begins shortly after S_1, peaks in midsystole, and does not quite extend to S_2 is descriptive of a(n):
   - **a.** early systolic murmur
   - **c.** late systolic murmur
   - **b.** midsystolic murmur
   - **d.** pansystolic murmur

ANSWERS TO SELF-LEARNING "UNKNOWN" HEART SOUNDS

1. Early systolic murmur

2. Midsystolic murmur

3. Pansystolic murmur

4. Late systolic murmur

5. Blowing quality

ANSWERS TO SELF-LEARNING QUESTIONS

1. a

2. b

3. d

4. c

5. b

8

Diastolic Murmurs

LEARNING OBJECTIVES

After reading this chapter, listening to the accompanying audio program, answering the self-learning questions at the end of the chapter, and listening to the "unknowns" on the audio program, the learner will be able to:

1. Define a diastolic murmur.
2. Identify the mechanisms of diastolic murmur production.
3. Identify the characteristics of an early diastolic, middiastolic, late diastolic, and pandiastolic murmur.
4. Differentiate between an early diastolic, middiastolic, late diastolic, and pandiastolic murmur.
5. Identify common adult abnormalities having diastolic murmurs.
6. Differentiate between systolic and diastolic murmurs.

Diastolic murmurs are sustained noises that are audible between S_2 and the next S_1. Unlike systolic murmurs, diastolic murmurs usually should be considered pathological and not normal.

MECHANISMS OF PRODUCTION

The three main mechanisms of **diastolic murmur** production are:
1. Aortic or pulmonic valve incompetence. During ventricular diastole, the pressure in the ventricles is less than that in the aorta or the pulmonary artery. If the aortic or pulmonic valves are incompetent, blood regurgitates back into the ventricles. The sustained noise of this regurgitation is the diastolic murmur.
2. Mitral stenosis or tricuspid stenosis. During the rapid filling phase of ventricular diastole, if the blood is forced into the ventricles through stenotic valves, a diastolic murmur occurs.
3. Increased blood flow across mitral or tricuspid valves. If volume or velocity of blood flow across the mitral or tricuspid valves is increased during ventricular diastole, a diastolic murmur occurs.

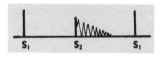

EARLY DIASTOLIC MURMURS

An early diastolic murmur begins with S_2 and peaks in the first third of diastole. This makes S_2 difficult to hear, whereas S_1 is easily heard. It usually is a regurgitant murmur with backward flow through an incompetent valve. Common causes are aortic regurgitation and pulmonic regurgitation.

 Listen now to a heart rate of 60 beats per minute. An early diastolic murmur will be added that is high in frequency and blowing in quality.

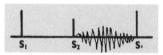

MIDDIASTOLIC MURMURS

A middiastolic murmur begins after S_2 and peaks in middiastole. (Both S_2 and S_1 are heard clearly.) Common causes are mitral stenosis and tricuspid stenosis. The murmur is low in frequency and rumbling in quality.

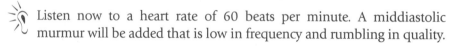 Listen now to a heart rate of 60 beats per minute. A middiastolic murmur will be added that is low in frequency and rumbling in quality.

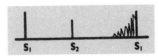

LATE DIASTOLIC MURMURS

A late diastolic murmur begins in the latter half of diastole, peaks in the later third of diastole, and extends to S_1. (S_2 is heard clearly; S_1 is difficult to hear.) It is known also as a *presystolic murmur.* It is commonly a component of the murmur of mitral stenosis or tricuspid stenosis. The late diastolic murmur is low in frequency and rumbling in quality.

 Listen now to a heart rate of 60 beats per minute. A late diastolic murmur will be added that is low in frequency and rumbling in quality. Listen next to a heart rate of 60 beats per minute. A middiastolic and a late diastolic murmur will be added that are low in frequency and rumbling in quality.

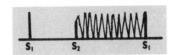

PANDIASTOLIC MURMURS

A pandiastolic murmur begins with S_2 and extends throughout the diastolic period. (Both S_2 and S_1 are difficult to hear.) Patent ductus arteriosus, the prototype of aorticopulmonary connections, is a classic example of this murmur. This condition is unusual in an adult, since it usually is corrected in childhood. It usually is best heard at base left and has both a systolic and a diastolic component. It is therefore known as a *continuous murmur.* It may be best heard with the bell chestpiece.

 Listen next to a heart rate of 60 beats per minute. A pandiastolic murmur will be added that is low in frequency and rumbling in quality.

For a review of the common adult abnormalities having diastolic murmurs, see Figure 8-1.

CLINICAL CORRELATION

To gain skill in listening to diastolic murmurs, seek out patients in whom these murmurs already have been identified. Common pathologic conditions in which this type of murmur is heard are mitral stenosis, tricuspid stenosis, aortic regurgitation, and pulmonic regurgitation. Initially, try to determine whether the murmur is in diastole or in systole. Also determine (1) location, (2) loudness, (3) frequency, (4) quality, and (5) radiation. Practice differentiating systolic from diastolic murmurs. Also

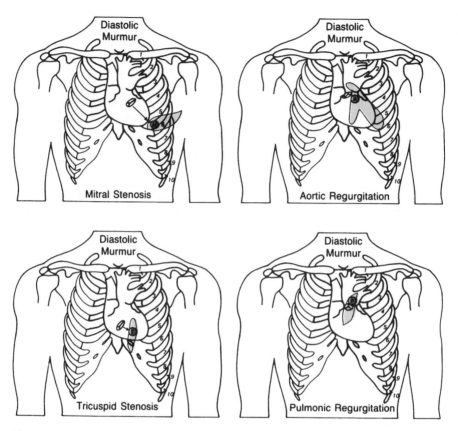

Figure 8-1   Common cardiac abnormalities with diastolic murmur(s). Area where murmur is heard best is *circled*; area of usual radiation is *shaded*.

practice recording the diastolic murmur on an auscultogram. In addition, write a narrative description of the diastolic murmur heard.

In a patient with a murmur of mitral stenosis, you may be able to hear the murmur by first finding the point of maximal impulse (PMI). Mark the PMI with a finger, and then place the bell of the stethoscope lightly over this area. The typical rumble of mitral stenosis may be heard. It may be inaudible when the stethoscope is moved out of this spot. The murmur can be brought out by having the patient cough several times (a mild exercise) or simply by the exertion of the patient turning to the left lateral position. (S_3 from the left ventricle also may be heard at this identical point and by using the same maneuvers.)

Some aortic diastolic murmurs may be heard along the right sternal border (third and fourth intercostal spaces [3 ICS and 4 ICS]). The development of aortic regurgitation with the murmur along the right sternal border (normally heard at Erb's point on the left sternal border) in a patient with a preexistent diastolic hypertension may be an indication of aortic aneurysm or dissection, or both.

SELF-LEARNING "UNKNOWN" HEART SOUNDS

 On the audio program, listen to the "unknown" heart sounds and identify the sound. Compare your answers with the answer key at the end of the chapter. Relisten to the audio program as needed to achieve mastery of the content.

Listen to the following diastolic murmurs.

1. Is the murmur early diastolic, middiastolic, late diastolic, or pandiastolic in nature?

2. Is the murmur early diastolic, middiastolic, late diastolic, or pandiastolic in nature?

3. Is the murmur early diastolic, middiastolic, late diastolic, or pandiastolic in nature?

4. Is the murmur early diastolic, middiastolic, late diastolic, or pandiastolic in nature?

5. What is the quality of this middiastolic murmur?

SELF-LEARNING QUESTIONS

Select the letter of the correct response. Compare your answers with the answer key at the end of the chapter. Reread the chapter as needed to achieve mastery of the content.

1. Sustained noises that are audible between S_2 and S_1 are:
   a. systolic murmur
   b. diastolic murmur
   c. ejection sound
   d. friction rub

2. Regurgitant blood flow across which valves will cause a diastolic murmur?
   a. mitral and aortic
   b. mitral and tricuspid
   c. tricuspid and pulmonic
   d. pulmonic and aortic

3. Forward blood flow across which abnormal valves will cause a diastolic murmur?

   a. mitral and aortic   **b.** mitral and tricuspid

   c. tricuspid and pulmonic   **d.** pulmonic and aortic

4. Common adult abnormalities having a diastolic murmur include:

   a. mitral stenosis and aortic regurgitation

   b. mitral stenosis and aortic stenosis

   c. mitral insufficiency and aortic insufficiency

   d. mitral insufficiency and aortic stenosis

5. A murmur that begins with S_2 and peaks in the first third of diastole is a(n):

   a. early diastolic murmur   **b.** middiastolic murmur

   c. late diastolic murmur   **d.** pandiastolic murmur

ANSWERS TO SELF-LEARNING "UNKNOWN" HEART SOUNDS

1. Middiastolic murmur

2. Early diastolic murmur

3. Late diastolic murmur

4. Pandiastolic murmur

5. Rumble quality

ANSWERS TO SELF-LEARNING QUESTIONS

1. b

2. d

3. b

4. a

5. a

9

Sounds Around S_1

LEARNING OBJECTIVES

After reading this chapter, listening to the accompanying audio program, answering the self-learning questions at the end of the chapter, and listening to the "unknowns" on the audio program, the learner will be able to:

1. Differentiate a normal split S_1 (M_1T_1) from a wide split S_1 (M_1T_1).
2. Differentiate a pulmonic ejection sound from an aortic ejection sound.
3. Identify the characteristics of a midsystolic click.
4. Identify:
   a. normal split S_1
   b. wide split S_1
   c. ejection sound—aortic or pulmonic
   d. midsystolic click
   e. S_4

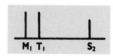

WIDE SPLIT S₁

An abnormal split S₁ may result from either electrical or mechanical causes. The resulting asynchrony of the ventricles causes the mitral and tricuspid valve closure sounds to be duration of 0.04 to 0.05 second apart, compared with the normal split S₁ of 0.02 second. The resulting sound is known as a *wide split S₁*. The wide split S₁ results when the physiologic split is augmented by conditions that delay tricuspid closure. Electrical causes include conduction problems such as right bundle branch block, ventricular premature beats (especially left), ventricular tachycardia, third-degree heart block with idioventricular rhythm, and, in some, pacing rhythms. The wide fixed splitting of S₁ seen in complete right bundle branch block is from delayed tricuspid closure resulting from the delay in stimulation. In ventricular premature contractions and ventricular tachycardia, the asynchronous contraction of the ventricles results in the wide split S₁. Mechanical delays in mitral or tricuspid closure that may cause wide splitting of S₁ include mitral stenosis, Ebstein's anomaly, and right or left atrial myxomas. The wide split S₁ is best heard at the left lateral sternal border (LLSB).

 Listen to a wide split S₁ as compared with a normal split S₁ and a single S₁.

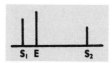

EJECTION SOUNDS

Ejection sounds are high-frequency "clicking" sounds that occur very shortly after the S₁. They usually are heard at either base right or base left. These sounds may be of either aortic or pulmonic origin and are produced when blood is ejected from the right ventricle or left ventricle either through a stenotic valve or into a dilated chamber. Because they are high in frequency, they are best heard with a diaphragm applied firmly.

Pulmonic ejection sounds are best heard at base left but may be heard anywhere along the LLSB (Figure 9-1, A). This sound may increase with expiration and decrease with inspiration in a patient with pulmonary stenosis. The exact reason for this respiratory variation is unknown. It may relate to pressure/volume changes between the right ventricle and pulmonary artery with respiration or be caused by the stenosed pulmonary valve opening with a "snap."

Besides being heard in pulmonic stenosis, pulmonic ejection sounds may be heard also in pulmonary hypertension, atrial septal defect,

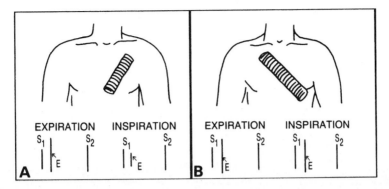

Figure 9-1   Area for auscultating ejection sounds (E) and respiratory effect. **A,** *Pulmonic ejection sound (E),* which decreases in intensity with inspiration and increases in intensity with expiration. **B,** *Aortic ejection sound (E),* which is not affected by respiration. (Modified with permission from Caccamo L, Erickson B: *Cardiac auscultation,* Youngstown, Ohio, 1975, St. Elizabeth's Hospital Medical Center.)

pulmonary embolism, and hyperthyroidism and in conditions causing enlargement of the pulmonary artery.

 Listen now to a pulmonic ejection sound compared to a single S$_1$.

Aortic ejection sounds are best heard at the apex but may be heard anywhere on a straight line from base right to the apex. This sound is not affected by respiration. It is heard in valvular aortic stenosis, aortic insufficiency, coarctation of the aorta, and aneurysm of the ascending aorta (see Figure 9-1, *B*).

 Listen now to an aortic ejection sound compared to a single S$_1$.

MIDSYSTOLIC CLICKS

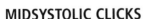
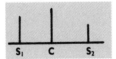

"Clicks" are high-frequency sounds that may be isolated or multiple sounds. Although the click usually occurs in the middle of systole, it may occur also in early or late systole. It occurs at least 0.14 second after S$_1$.

The most common cause of a midsystolic click or clicks is the ballooning of one of the mitral valve leaflets (usually the posterior one) into the left atrium at the point of maximal ventricular ejection. The click is heard when the chordae tendineae, which may be longer than normal, suddenly stop the ballooning leaflet. This is descriptive of mitral valve prolapse and is the most common cause of the midsystolic click.

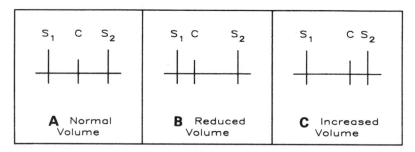

Figure 9-2   Correlation of click's *(C)* distance to S$_1$ and ventricular volume. **A,** *Normal* ventricular volume (click in *mid*systole). **B,** *Reduced* ventricular volume (click is *closer* to S$_1$). **C,** *Increased* ventricular volume (click is *farther* from S$_1$).

Because the clicks usually are of mitral valve origin, they are best heard at the apex. They may be heard also toward the left lateral sternal border when the posterior leaflet is primarily involved.

 Listen now to a midsystolic click compared to a single S$_1$.

Factors that reduce ventricular volume (standing, Valsalva, tachycardia, amyl nitrite) will cause the click to move closer to S$_1$. With reduced ventricular volume, the mitral valve closes earlier after the S$_1$ and therefore the click moves closer to S$_1$.

 Listen now to a midsystolic click that moves closer to S$_1$ with standing.

Factors that increase ventricular volume (squatting, bradycardia, propranolol, vasopressors) will cause the click to move farther from S$_1$. With increased ventricular volume, mitral valve closure occurs later and the click therefore moves farther from S$_1$ (Figure 9-2).

 Listen now to a midsystolic click that moves farther from S$_1$ with squatting.

For a summary of the various sounds that can occur around S$_1$ and a method of differentiating one from the other, see Table 9-1.

CLINICAL CORRELATION

The stethoscope is still the best instrument to detect and diagnose a prolapse of the mitral valve that occurs in as many as 15 million Americans. Careful listening is necessary to hear the click and the late

TABLE 9-1
Differential for Sounds Around the First Heart Sound (S$_1$)

Sound Heard	Area Heard Loudest	Respiratory Variation	Chestpiece	Change With Pressure on Bell	Listen at Base Right S$_1$ Split?	Listen at Base Right S$_2$ Split?
Normal split	LLSB	↑Slight inspiration	D	None	No	Normal
Wide split	LLSB	↑Inspiration	D	None	No	Wide
S$_4$ right	LLSB	↑Inspiration	B	Decrease	No	Normal
S$_4$ left	Apex	↓Inspiration ↑Expiration	B	Decrease	No	Normal
Ejection pulmonic	Base left	↓Inspiration ↑Expiration	D	None	Yes	Wide
Ejection aortic	Apex	None	D	None	Yes	Wide

Modified with permission from Caccamo L, Erickson B: *Cardiac auscultation*, Youngstown, Ohio, 1975, St. Elizabeth's Hospital Medical Center.
LLSB, Left lateral sternal border; *D*, diaphragm; *B*, bell.

systolic murmur (see Chapter 10) that are typically transient, intermittent, and varying. Heart disease in mitral valve prolapse is more commonly absent than present, and the majority of individuals with the syndrome are asymptomatic. Because individuals with mitral valve prolapse have increased risk of developing infective endocarditis after invasive procedures, prophylactic antibiotics are recommended before dental procedures (including cleaning, filling, and extractions), surgical procedures, and invasive procedures of the gastrointestinal and genitourinary tracts.

In the clinical setting, pay particular attention to S_1 and to "sounds around the first sound." Can you differentiate a normal split S_1 from a wide split S_1; from a midsystolic click; from ejection sounds—aortic or pulmonic; from S_4? Use Table 9-1 to help you in your differentiation.

SELF-LEARNING "UNKNOWN" HEART SOUNDS

 On the audio program, listen to the "unknown" heart sounds and identify the sound. Compare your answers with the answer key at the end of the chapter. Relisten to the audio program as needed to achieve mastery of the content.

You are listening to the heart at base left with the diaphragm applied firmly:

   1. Is S_1 a normal split S_1 or a wide split S_1?

You are listening to a heart with the diaphragm applied firmly:
    At the LLSB, what do you hear?
    At the apex, what do you hear?
    At base right, what do you hear?
    At base left, what do you hear?

   2. The sound you hear around S_1 is a(n):
    a. normal split S_1 **b.** wide split S_1
    c. aortic ejection sound   **d.** pulmonic ejection sound

You are listening to a heart with the diaphragm pressed firmly:
    At the LLSB, what do you hear?
    At the apex, what do you hear?
    At base right, what do you hear?
    At base left, what do you hear?

3. The sound you hear around S$_1$ is a(n):
   a. normal split S$_1$
   b. wide split S$_1$
   c. aortic ejection sound
   d. pulmonic ejection sound

You are listening to a heart with the diaphragm applied firmly:
   At the LLSB, what do you hear?
   At the apex, what do you hear?
   At the base right, what do you hear?
   At base left, what do you hear?

4. The sound you hear around S$_1$ is a(n):
   a. normal split S$_1$
   b. wide split S$_1$
   c. aortic ejection sound
   d. midsystolic click

You are listening to the heart at the apex:
   Using the bell lightly held, what do you hear?
   Using the bell firmly pressed, what do you hear?
   Using the diaphragm, what do you hear?

5. The sound you hear around S$_1$ is a(n):
   a. normal split S$_1$
   b. aortic ejection sound
   c. S$_4$
   d. midsystolic click

SELF-LEARNING QUESTIONS

Select the letter of the correct response. Compare your answers with the answer key at the end of the chapter. Reread the chapter as needed to achieve mastery of the content.

1. In right bundle branch block or ventricular tachycardia, which of the following will be heard?
   a. normal split S$_1$
   b. wide split S$_1$
   c. pulmonic ejection sound
   d. midsystolic click

2. A high-frequency sound that occurs very shortly after S$_1$ and is heard anywhere on a straight line from base right to the apex is descriptive of a(n):
   a. wide split S$_1$
   b. midsystolic click
   c. aortic ejection sound
   d. pulmonic ejection sound

3. In a midsystolic click, factors that reduce ventricular volume will cause the click to:

    a. disappear   **b.** become louder
    c. move farther from S_1 **d.** move closer to S_1

4. A wide split S_1 is best heard at:
    a. base right   **b.** base left
    c. apex   **d.** left lateral sternal border

5. A midsystolic click is best heard at
    a. base right   **b.** base left
    c. apex   **d.** left lateral sternal border

ANSWERS TO SELF-LEARNING "UNKNOWN" HEART SOUNDS

1. Wide split S_1

2. c

3. d

4. d

5. c

ANSWERS TO SELF-LEARNING QUESTIONS

1. b

2. c

3. d

4. d

5. c

C·H·A·P·T·E·R

10

Sounds Around S_2

LEARNING OBJECTIVES

After reading this chapter, listening to the accompanying audio program, answering the self-learning questions at the end of the chapter, and listening to the "unknowns" on the audio program, the learner will be able to:

1. Identify the characteristics of a paradoxical split S_2.
2. Identify the characteristics of a wide split S_2.
3. Identify the characteristics of a fixed split S_2.
4. Identify the characteristics of a narrow split S_2.
5. Identify:
   a. physiological split S_2
   b. paradoxical split S_2
   c. wide split S_2
   d. fixed split S_2
   e. narrow split S_2
   f. S_3
   g. opening snap

PARADOXICAL SPLIT S₂

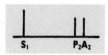

If the closure of the aortic valve is delayed, there may be a reversal of normal closure sequence of S_2, with pulmonic closure (P_2) occurring before aortic closure (A_2) (Figure 10-1). Paradoxical splitting of S_2 is never heard in the absence of a heart abnormality.

A paradoxical split S_2 is identified clinically when during inspiration there is a single S_2 and during expiration a split S_2. Paradoxical, or reversed, splitting of S_2 may occur with marked volume or pressure loads on the left ventricle (severe aortic stenosis, severe aortic regurgitation, and large patent ductus arteriosus). With the increased volume in the left ventricle, ventricular emptying is delayed, thus delaying closure of the aortic valve. It also occurs in conduction defects that delay left ventricular depolarization (complete left bundle branch block). Conduction defects that delay left ventricular depolarization also delay left ventricular emptying, thus also delaying closure of the aortic valve.

 Listen now to a paradoxical split S_2—split audible on expiration; single on inspiration.

WIDE SPLIT S₂

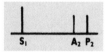

The normal physiological split S_2 can be accentuated by conditions that cause abnormal delay in pulmonic valve closure. Five such conditions are:

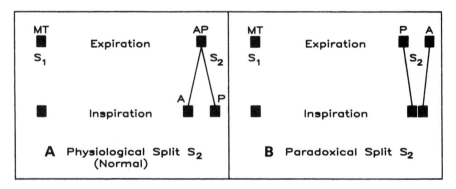

Figure 10-1   Splitting of the second heart sound (S_2). **A**, Physiological split S_2, which splits on *inspiration*, is compared with **B**, paradoxical split S_2, which splits on *expiration*. *M*, Mitral; *T*, tricuspid; *A*, aortic closure; *AP*, aortic pulmonic closure; *P*, pulmonic closure. (Reproduced with permission from Caccamo L, Erickson B: *Cardiac auscultation*, Youngstown, Ohio, 1975, St. Elizabeth's Hospital Medical Center.)

1. Increased volume in right ventricle as compared with the left (atrial septal defect, ventricular septal defect)
2. Chronic outflow tract obstruction to the right ventricle (pulmonary stenosis)
3. Acute or chronic dilation of the right ventricle caused by sudden rise in pulmonary artery pressure (pulmonary embolism)
4. Electrical delay or activation of right ventricle (complete right bundle branch block)
5. Decreased elastic recoil of pulmonary artery (idiopathic dilation of the pulmonary artery)

Early closure of the aortic valve also may contribute to a wide split S₂. Mitral insufficiency may cause early closure of the aortic valve, since some of the left ventricular output is regurgitated into the atrium.

The wide split has a duration of 0.04 to 0.05 second. The physiological (normal) split is 0.03 second (Figure 10-2, *A*).

Listen now to a wide split S₂. Compare it to a normal split S₂ and a single S₂.

FIXED SPLIT S₂

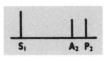

A split that does not change its width with inspiration or expiration is called a *fixed split* (see Figure 10-2, *B*). It occurs when the ventricles are

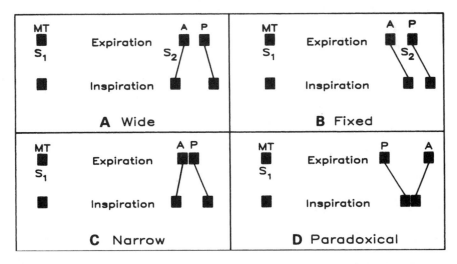

Figure 10-2   Splitting of the second heart sound (S₂). **A**, Wide. **B**, Fixed. **C**, Narrow. **D**, Paradoxical. *M*, Mitral; *T*, tricuspid; *A*, aortic closure; *AP*, aortic pulmonic closure; *P*, pulmonic closure. (Reproduced with permission from Caccamo L, Erickson B: *Cardiac auscultation*, Youngstown, Ohio, 1975, St. Elizabeth's Hospital Medical Center.)

unable to change their volumes with respiration. This can occur in congestive heart failure, cardiomyopathy, atrial septal defect, or ventricular septal defect. In congestive heart failure the congested lungs cannot withhold much blood from the left ventricle during inspiration; thus left ventricular volume is not markedly affected by respiration. Another factor is that a dilated and poorly compliant left ventricle, which is common in congestive failure or cardiomyopathy, may not be able to respond to small changes in volume. Atrial septal defect or ventricular septal defect may prevent the left ventricle alone from changing size on respiration, or there may be a selective shortening of the left ventricular ejection time with an early aortic closure, as in severe mitral insufficiency or ventricular septal defect.

 Listen now to a fixed split S_2. Compare it to a physiological split S_2.

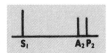

NARROW SPLIT S_2

A narrow split S_2 may be heard in conditions that cause increased left ventricular volume without markedly affecting the right side (uncomplicated patent ductus arteriosus with aortic regurgitation). It also may be heard in conditions causing obstruction to outflow of the left ventricle (aortic stenosis or electrical delay, as in left bundle branch block). The conditions just mentioned would cause delay in the closure of the aortic valve but would not delay closure of the pulmonic valve (A_2 closer to P_2).

With aging, the pulmonary component comes earlier and the split narrows. This occurs because there is less blood pooling in the lungs (A_2 closer to P_2) and less venous return (P_2 closer to A_2) (see Figure 10-2, C).

 Listen to a narrow split S_2. Compare it to a physiological split S_2.

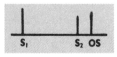

OPENING SNAP

Normally the opening of the mitral valve is not discernible, but under certain conditions the opening is audible and becomes known as the *opening snap*—a short, high-frequency click or snap that occurs after the second S_2. It is the result of an audible opening of the mitral valve resulting from stiffening (mitral stenosis) or increased flow (ventricular septal defect or patent ductus arteriosus). It is best heard between the apex and the left lateral sternal border (LLSB) with the diaphragm applied firmly. During inspiration the opening snap is softer (because of decreased blood return to the left ventricle). With increased tricuspid flow, as in atrial septal defect, a tricuspid opening snap may be heard. It is a high-frequency sound heard loudest at the LLSB with the diaphragm applied firmly. The tricuspid opening snap becomes louder with inspiration.

The opening snap is one of the early signs of mitral stenosis, and initially the opening snap is widely separated from S_2 (making it easy to hear). As the left atrial pressure increases, the opening of the mitral valve occurs earlier in diastole; therefore the opening snap moves closer to S_2. (You may then confuse it with a split S_2. However, the opening snap is of higher frequency and more "clicky" than S_2.) In severe stenosis the opening snap may merge with the components of S_2.

 Listen now to an S_2 followed by an opening snap.

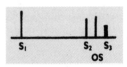

DIFFERENTIATING S_3 FROM THE OPENING SNAP

The opening snap occurs earlier after S_2 and is a high-frequency sound best heard with the diaphragm applied firmly. S_3 occurs later than the opening snap, following S_2 and is a low-frequency sound best heard with the bell held lightly. For a synopsis of the various sounds that can occur around the S_2 and a method of differentiating one from the other, see Table 10-1.

 Listen now to an S_3 and differentiate if from an opening snap.

CLINICAL CORRELATION

In the clinical setting, pay particular attention to S_2 and the "sounds around the second sound." Can you differentiate a physiological split S_2 from a paradoxical split S_2; from a wide split S_2; from a fixed split S_2; from a narrow split S_2; from S_3; from an opening snap? Use Table 10-1 to help you in your differentiation.

A technique taught by Harvey can be used to develop and sharpen your ability to detect degrees of splitting. Use your knuckles or fingers and strike two knuckles or fingers against a hard surface. By varying the degree of asynchrony, you can accurately simulate degrees of splitting from close to wide. If you use only one knuckle or finger, a single sound

TABLE 10-1
Differential for Sounds Around the Second Heart Sound (S₂)

Sound Heard	Area Heard Loudest	Respiratory Variation	Chestpiece	Change With Pressure on Bell
Normal split	Base left	Heard on inspiration	D	No
Wide split	Base left	Heard on inspiration	D	No
Fixed split	Base left	None	D	No
Narrow split	Base left	Heard on inspiration	D	No
Paradoxical split	Base left	Heard on expiration	D	No
Opening snap	Apex or LLSB	↓Inspiration ↑Expiration	D	No
S₄ right	Xiphoid or LLSB	↑Inspiration	B	Yes
S₄ left	Apex	↓Inspiration ↑Expiration	B	Yes

Modified with permission from Caccamo L, Erickson B: *Cardiac auscultation*, Youngstown, Ohio, 1975, St. Elizabeth's Hospital Medical Center.
LLSB, Left lateral sternal border; *D*, diaphragm; *B*, bell.

is simulated. (This same technique can be used to simulate S₁, S₂, S₃, S₄, or an opening snap.)

SELF-LEARNING "UNKNOWN" HEART SOUNDS

 On the audio program, listen to the "unknown" heart sounds and identify the sound. Compare your answers with the answer key at the end of the chapter. Relisten to the audio program as needed to achieve mastery of the content.

You are listening to the heart at base left with the diaphragm applied firmly:

1. Is the S₂ splitting physiologically or paradoxically?

2. Is the S₂ splitting physiologically or paradoxically?

3. Is S₂ a wide or a narrow split?

You are listening to the heart at the apex:
   Using the bell held lightly, what do you hear?

Using the bell applied firmly, what do you hear?
Using the diaphragm applied firmly, what do you hear?

4. Is there an S$_3$ or a wide split S$_2$?

You are listening to the heart at the apex:
Using the bell held lightly, what do you hear?
Using the bell applied firmly, what do you hear?
Using the diaphragm applied firmly, what do you hear?

5. Is there an S$_3$ or an opening snap?

SELF-LEARNING QUESTIONS

Select the letter of the correct response. Compare your answers with the answer key at the end of the chapter. Reread the chapter as needed to achieve mastery of the content.

1. The reversal of the normal closure sequence of S$_2$ with the pulmonic closure (P$_2$) occurring before aortic closure (A$_2$) is descriptive of a:
   a. physiological split S$_2$
   b. paradoxical split S$_2$
   c. wide split S$_2$
   d. narrow split S$_2$

2. Abnormal delay in pulmonic valve closure (P$_2$) is descriptive of a:
   a. physiological split S$_2$
   b. paradoxical split S$_2$
   c. wide split S$_2$
   d. narrow split S$_2$

3. A split of S$_2$ that does not change its width with inspiration or expiration is descriptive of a:
   a. physiological split S$_2$
   b. paradoxical split S$_2$
   c. fixed split S$_2$
   d. narrow split S$_2$

4. A split of S$_2$ in which the pulmonic component (P$_2$) comes earlier than normal is descriptive of a:
   a. physiological split S$_2$
   b. paradoxical split S$_2$
   c. fixed split S$_2$
   d. narrow split S$_2$

5. A short, high-frequency sound that occurs after S$_2$ and is the result of the audible opening of the mitral valve as a result of stiffness is descriptive of a(n):
   a. physiological split S$_2$
   b. paradoxical split S$_2$
   c. fixed split S$_2$
   d. opening snap after S$_2$

ANSWERS TO SELF-LEARNING "UNKNOWN" HEART SOUNDS

1. Physiologically split S_2

2. Paradoxically split S_2

3. Wide split S_2

4. S_3

5. Opening snap

ANSWERS TO SELF-LEARNING QUESTIONS

1. b

2. c

3. c

4. b

5. d

11

Friction Rubs: Pericardial And Pleural

LEARNING OBJECTIVES

After reading this chapter, listening to the accompanying audio program, answering the self-learning questions at the end of the chapter, and listening to the "unknowns" on the audio program, the learner will be able to:

1. Identify the common causes of a pericardial friction rub.
2. Identify the auscultatory signs of a pericardial friction rub.
3. Identify the sound characteristics of a pericardial friction rub.
4. Identify the common causes of a pleural friction rub.
5. Identify the auscultatory signs of a pleural friction rub.
6. Identify the sound characteristics of a pleural friction rub.
7. Differentiate a pericardial friction rub from a pleural friction rub.

To differentiate between pericardial and pleural friction rubs, the listener must consider the following factors.

PERICARDIAL FRICTION RUBS

Causes

A pericardial friction rub is a sign of pericardial inflammation. Some common etiological factors are:

1. **Infective pericarditis.** Many organisms may cause infective pericarditis, including viral, pyogenic, tubercular, and mycotic.
2. **Noninfective pericarditis.** Myocardial infarction, uremia, neoplasms, myxedema, open heart surgery, and trauma are some of the noninfective causes of a pericardial friction rub.
3. **Autoimmune problems.** Rheumatic fever, collagen vascular disease, drug-induced (e.g., procainamide) injury, and postmyocardial injury (Dressler's syndrome) are autoimmune causes of pericardial friction rub.

Auscultatory Signs

The auscultatory signs of a pericardial friction rub are **one systolic** sound and **two diastolic** sounds. The systolic sound (between S_1 and S_2) may occur anywhere in systole. The two diastolic sounds occur at the times the ventricles are stretched in diastole:

1. In early diastole near the end of the early diastolic filling. (This is the same time that an S_3 would occur.)
2. At end diastole, when atrial contraction produces sudden ventricular expansion. (This is the same time that an S_4 would occur.) If atrial contraction does not occur, as in atrial fibrillation, the second diastolic sound is not heard.

Sound Characteristics

1. The pericardial friction rub has a scratching, grating, or squeaking to-and-fro leathery quality.
2. This rub is high in frequency and therefore best heard with the diaphragm chestpiece applied firmly.
3. The pericardial friction rub tends to be louder during inspiration. This may be a result of:
   a. The downward pull of the diaphragm on the pericardium during inspiration, which causes the pericardium to be drawn more tautly over the heart during inspiration
   b. The expanded lung pressing on the pericardium

c. The fact that the pericardium is stretched more during inspiration than during expiration because the expansion of the right ventricle is greater during inspiration than that of the left ventricle during expiration

4. The pericardial friction rub may be most audible in some patients during **forced expiration** with the patient leaning forward or on hands and knees. (These maneuvers cause less air to be between the pericardium and the stethoscope and also bring the heart closer to the chest wall.)

5. The pericardial friction rub is likely to be transitory or inconstant. This means that it comes and goes suddenly.

6. The pericardial friction rub may be heard anywhere on the pericardium, but it is often loudest at the left lateral sternal border (LLSB).

7. Most patients with a pericardial friction rub also have a tachycardia.

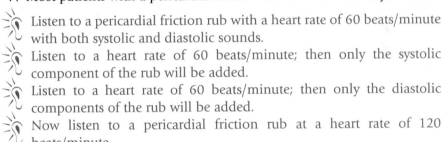

Listen to a pericardial friction rub with a heart rate of 60 beats/minute with both systolic and diastolic sounds.

Listen to a heart rate of 60 beats/minute; then only the systolic component of the rub will be added.

Listen to a heart rate of 60 beats/minute; then only the diastolic components of the rub will be added.

Now listen to a pericardial friction rub at a heart rate of 120 beats/minute.

Listen to a real heart with a pericardial friction rub; all three components are present.

PLEURAL FRICTION RUBS

Causes

A pleural friction rub is a sign of pleural inflammation and indicates that the visceral and parietal surfaces of the pleura are rubbing together. Some common etiological factors of pleural friction rubs are:

1. Pneumonia
2. Viral infections
3. Tuberculosis
4. Pulmonary embolism

Auscultatory Signs

The auscultatory signs of a pleural friction rub are **one sound during inspiration** and **one sound during expiration** (this may not always be heard).

Sound Characteristics

1. The pleural friction rub has a grating or creaking sound similar to that heard in the pericardial friction rub.
2. This rub is high in frequency and therefore is best heard with the diaphragm chestpiece applied firmly.
3. The pleural friction rub is heard during inspiration and sometimes during expiration.
4. The pleural friction rub commonly is heard in the lower anterolateral chest wall (the area of greatest thoracic mobility) on the side of the pleural inflammation.
5. The pleural friction rub decreases with a decrease in lung movement. The sound disappears if the breath is held.
6. The pleural friction rub has a superficial character. It sounds closer to the surface than does a pericardial friction rub.

 Listen to a pleural friction rub in a real individual. Note the inspiratory and expiratory components.

Compare the pleural friction rub to a pericardial friction rub. First a pleural friction rub, then a pericardial friction rub.

TABLE 11-1
Summary for Differentiating Pericardial From Pleural Friction Rubs

	Pericardial	Pleural
Frequency	High	High
Quality	Scratching, grating, squeaking	Grating or creaking
Chestpiece best heard with	Diaphragm	Diaphragm
Timing	One systolic sound; two diastolic sounds	One sound on inspiration; one sound on expiration (this may be absent)
	Transitory	Transitory (but less abrupt)
Site	Over pericardium (left chest)	Over anterolateral chest—right or left side
Respiratory variant	Louder during inspiration	Decreases with decrease in breathing; gone when breath held
Surface proximity	Farther from surface	Superficial; closer to surface

CLINICAL CORRELATION

In the clinical setting seek out patients with pericardial and pleural friction rubs. Use Table 11-1 to help you in your differentiation. Compare the sounds of the friction rubs with those of systolic and diastolic murmurs. Practice charting your findings. If you have difficulty differentiating a pericardial friction rub from a pleural friction rub, ask the patient to stop breathing. (It is a good idea to hold your own breath at the same time so that you remember to permit the patient to again breathe.) If during respiratory cessation the sound goes away, it is a pleural rub; if the sound remains, it is a pericardial rub.

SELF-LEARNING "UNKNOWN" HEART SOUNDS

 On the audio program, listen to the "unknown" heart sounds and identify the sound. Compare your answers with the answer key at the end of the chapter. Relisten to the audio program as needed to achieve mastery of the content.

You are listening at the LLSB. You hear the following sound.

1. You identify the sound as a:
   a. pericardial friction rub   b. pleural friction rub
   c. systolic murmur   d. diastolic murmur

You are listening at the apex. You hear the following sound.

2. You identify the sound as a:
   a. pericardial friction rub   b. pleural friction rub
   c. systolic murmur   d. diastolic murmur

SELF-LEARNING QUESTIONS

Select the letter of the correct response, or provide requested information. Compare your answers with the answer key at the end of the chapter. Reread the chapter as needed to achieve mastery of the content.

1. Identify two of the common etiological factors of a pericardial friction rub.
   a.
   b.

2. One of the diastolic sounds of the pericardial friction rub occurs in early diastole; the other occurs at:
   a. middiastole
   b. late diastole
   c. rapid diastolic filling
   d. none of the above

3. Identify two of the common etiological factors of a pleural friction rub in early diastole.
   a.
   b.

4. Which characteristic is most helpful in differentiating a pericardial from a pleural friction rub?
   a. quality
   b. frequency
   c. breath-holding
   d. site

ANSWERS TO SELF-LEARNING "UNKNOWN" HEART SOUNDS

1. a

2. b

ANSWERS TO SELF-LEARNING QUESTIONS

1. Any two of the following:
   Infective (e.g., viral, tuberculosis)
   Noninfective (e.g., myocardial infarction)
   Autoimmune (rheumatic fever)

2. b

3. Any two of the following:
   Pneumonia
   Viral infections
   Tuberculosis
   Pulmonary embolism

4. c

12

Prosthetic Valve Sounds

LEARNING OBJECTIVES

After reading this chapter, listening to the accompanying audio program, answering the self-learning questions at the end of the chapter, and listening to the "unknowns" on the audio program, the learner will be able to:

1. Name two categories of prosthetic heart valves.
2. Identify the types of prosthetic heart valves with fewer thromboembolic complications.
3. Identify the heart sounds made by a caged-ball valve placed in the mitral or aortic position.
4. Identify the heart sounds made by a tilting-disk valve placed in the mitral or aortic position.
5. Identify the heart sounds made by a bileaflet valve placed in the mitral or aortic position.
6. Identify the heart sounds made by a porcine or bovine pericardial valve placed in the mitral or aortic position.

PROSTHETIC HEART VALVES

The two categories of prosthetic heart valves that are available today are *mechanical* and *biological.*

Mechanical heart valves have been used in humans since the early 1960s. These valves are made from a combination of metal alloys, pyrolytic carbon, and Dacron. Although their construction makes them very durable, it also makes them very vulnerable to thromboembolism. Patients with mechanical valves require anticoagulation. Because mechanical valves are more durable, they may be selected for use in young people who have a longer life expectancy.

Biological heart valves tend to be the less durable of the two varieties but have less thromboembolic complications and therefore offer freedom from anticoagulation. Because of the valves' decreased longevity, they may be chosen for use in patients older than 65 years who have a shorter life expectancy. They also are the valves of choice for patients in whom anticoagulation is contraindicated or for patients who are known to be noncompliant with drug therapy.

The sounds generated by prosthetic valves depend on the type of valve used, the area in which the prosthesis is placed, and whether the valve is functioning normally or abnormally. Each type has advantages and disadvantages, and each has distinctive sounds and murmurs. A review of valve types follows.

After reading this chapter, consider how a prosthetic valve would change the first and second heart sounds.

MECHANICAL PROSTHETIC VALVES

The three commonly used types of mechanical valves that are placed in the mitral or aortic position are the *caged-ball, tilting-disk,* and *bileaflet* (Figure 12-1).

Caged-Ball Valve

As the name implies, the **caged-ball valve** consists of a ball that moves freely within a three- or four-sided metallic cage mounted on a circular sewing ring. Blood flows through the cage and around the ball/poppet. Changes in chamber pressure cause the ball to move back and forth in its cage, opening and closing the valve. This type of valve has been in use for more than 40 years. It was the first durable mechanical valve and has an excellent record for being implanted for up to 20 years. The Starr-Edwards is the prototype of the caged-ball valve and is the most commonly used of its type in the United States today. Other types of the caged-ball valve

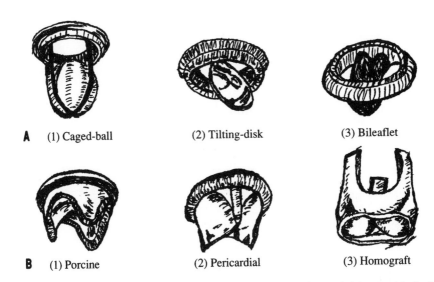

A   (1) Caged-ball   (2) Tilting-disk   (3) Bileaflet

B   (1) Porcine   (2) Pericardial   (3) Homograft

Figure 12-1   Common prosthetic heart valves. **A**, *Mechanical:* (1) caged-ball; (2) tilting-disk; (3) bileaflet. **B**, *Biological:* (1) porcine; (2) pericardial; (3) homograft.

include the Smeloff-Cutter, the McGovern-Cromie, and the DeBakey-Surgitool. The Smeloff-Cutter uses a double-cage design with three titanium struts on each of the inflow and outflow regions to contain the Silastic ball. The cages are open at the apex. The McGovern-Cromie valve is equipped with two rows of interlocking pins that are extended into the annulus. The DeBakey-Surgitool uses a pyrolytic carbon poppet intended to limit ball variance, which is a mechanical dysfunction of the prosthesis caused by physical and chemical changes in the Silastic poppets.

Caged-ball valves have a distinct, high-frequency, audible opening and closing sound that generally is described as "crisp" and "clicking" and may be audible at the bedside without the aid of a stethoscope. In the mitral or tricuspid position, a prominent opening click corresponds in timing to an opening snap. The closing sound coincides with the first heart sound. These sounds are best heard at the apex in the mitral position and at the left lateral sternal border (LLSB) in the tricuspid position. In the aortic position, there is a prominent opening click, which commonly obscures the first heart sound. When this valve is placed in the mitral or aortic position, an early "decrescendo" or systolic ejection murmur, grade 2/6 or 3/6, may be heard. The murmur is accentuated in conditions that augment the stroke volume. The presence of a diastolic murmur is considered abnormal.

 Listen now to a patient with a Starr-Edwards caged-ball valve.

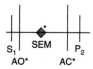

Aortic sounds:

*SEM, Systolic ejection murmur; AO, aortic opening; AC, aortic closing.

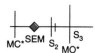

Mitral sounds:

*MC, Mitral closing; MO, mitral opening.

Tilting-Disk Valve

The **tilting-disk valve** is a free-floating, lens-shaped disk mounted on a circular sewing ring. Depending on the type, the disk tilts open anywhere from 60 degrees (Björk-Shiley valve) to 80 degrees (Lillehei-Kaster valve) to allow blood to flow through. The tilting-disk valve allows some amount of central flow and has a low profile that permits its use in the mitral position without compromising the left ventricular outflow tract. It does not have an audible opening sound in either the mitral or aortic position but does produce distinct closing sounds. Absence of these closing sounds is abnormal. An early systolic to midsystolic ejection murmur, grade 2/6, is common. When the valve is placed in the aortic position, the sounds are best heard at base right. When the valve is used in the mitral position, the sounds are best heard at the apex.

Aortic sounds:

* ⋮⋮⋮ = Sound not audible.

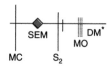

Mitral sounds:

*DM, Diastolic murmur.

Bileaflet Valve

The **bileaflet valve** is the newest of the commonly used valves including the St. Jude Medical valve. It has two semicircular leaflets mounted on a circular sewing ring that open in the center. The leaflets open at an angle of 85 degrees and close at an angle of 35 degrees. Blood flow is central, and since the valve has a low profile, it may be used in the mitral position. The bileaflet valve does not have an audible opening sound in either the mitral or aortic position but does produce a distinct closing sound. Absence of the closing sound is abnormal. A midsystolic ejection murmur is normal. In the aortic position, the sounds are best heard at base right. When the valve is placed in the mitral position, the sounds are best heard at the apex. When the valve is placed in the mitral position, a diastolic murmur similar to that found in mitral stenosis may be heard. The diastolic murmur is considered abnormal only if it changes or if a new diastolic murmur occurs.

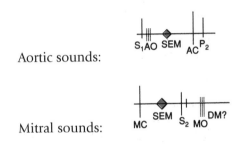

Aortic sounds: S_1AO SEM $_{AC}$$P_2$

Mitral sounds: MC   SEM S_2 MO   DM?

BIOLOGICAL PROSTHETIC VALVES

Biological valves may be classified as *allograft* (isograft) from the fascia lata of the pulmonic valve; *homologous* (allograft) from an aortic valve obtained from a corpse or dura mater; and *heterologous* (xenograft) from the bovine aortic valve, porcine aortic valve, or bovine pericardium (see Figure 12-1). The heterologous (xenograft) currently is the most extensively used of the biologic valves.

Porcine Heterograft

The **porcine heterograft** is a porcine valve mounted on a semiflexible stent and preserved with glutaraldehyde. Blood flows almost unobstructed through a central opening. Common types are the Hancock and the Carpentier-Edwards.

Bovine Pericardial Heterograft

The **bovine pericardial heterograft** is made from bovine pericardium fashioned into three identical cusps that are mounted on a cloth-covered frame (Ionescu-Shiley valve). Blood flow is unobstructed.

When used in the mitral position, porcine heterologous and bovine pericardial heterologous valves have crisp, high-pitched opening and closing sounds. These sounds are best heard at the apex and may be accompanied by systolic murmur or diastolic rumble. When the valves are implanted in the aortic position, opening sounds generally are not heard but closing sounds may be audible. A midsystolic murmur may be audible at the left lateral sternal border. A diastolic murmur would be considered abnormal.

Listen now to a patient with a porcine heart valve in the aortic position.

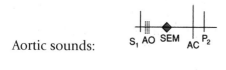

Aortic sounds: S_1 AO SEM AC P_2

Mitral sounds: MC SEM S_2 MO DM

SELF-LEARNING "UNKNOWN" HEART SOUNDS

On the audio program, listen to the "unknown" heart sounds and identify the sound. Compare your answers with the answer key at the end of the chapter. Relisten to the audio program as needed to achieve mastery of the content.

1. Is the sound made by a mechanical or biological valve?

2. Is the sound made by a mechanical or biological valve?

SELF-LEARNING QUESTIONS

Select the letter of the correct response, or provide requested information. Compare your answers with the answer key at the end of the chapter. Reread the chapter as needed to achieve mastery of the content.

1. Name the two categories of prosthetic heart valves.
   a.
   b.

2. The prosthetic heart valves with less thromboembolic complications are:
   a. Starr-Edwards and Björk-Shiley
   b. Starr-Edwards and bileaflet
   c. porcine and bovine pericardium
   d. porcine and Lillehei-Kaster

3. The sounds made by a caged-ball valve placed in the mitral position
include a systolic ejection murmur and:
   a. mitral opening and closing sounds
   b. mitral closing sound, with silent mitral opening
   c. mitral opening sound, with silent mitral closing
   d. silent mitral opening and closing sounds

4. The sounds made by a tilting-disk valve placed in the aortic position
include a systolic ejection murmur and:
   a. aortic opening and closing sounds
   b. aortic closing sound, with silent aortic opening
   c. aortic opening sound, with silent aortic closing
   d. silent aortic opening and closing sounds

5. The sounds made by a bileaflet valve placed in the aortic position
include a systolic ejection murmur and:
   a. aortic opening and closing sounds
   b. aortic closing sound, with silent aortic opening
   c. aortic opening sound, with silent aortic closing
   d. silent aortic opening and closing sounds

6. The sounds made by a porcine valve placed in the mitral position
include a systolic ejection murmur and:
   a. mitral opening and closing sounds
   b. silent mitral opening and closing sounds
   c. mitral opening sound
   d. mitral closing sound

ANSWERS TO SELF-LEARNING "UNKNOWN" HEART SOUNDS

1. Sound from mechanical valve

2. Sound from biological valve

ANSWERS TO SELF-LEARNING QUESTIONS

1. a. mechanical
   b. biological

2. c

3. a

4. b

5. b

6. a

13

Sounds After Heart Surgery and Other Sounds

LEARNING OBJECTIVES

After reading this chapter, listening to the accompanying audio program, answering the self-learning questions at the end of the chapter, and listening to the "unknowns" on the audio program, the learner will be able to:

1. Identify changes in normal heart sounds in a patient with an endocardial pacemaker.
2. Identify the cause of the pericardial knock.
3. Differentiate a sternal click from a midsystolic click.
4. Recognize the auscultatory findings of subcutaneous emphysema.
5. Recognize the auscultatory findings of an intraaortic balloon pump.
6. Recognize the auscultatory findings of intracardiac myxomas.

INTRAAORTIC BALLOON PUMP

The **intraaortic balloon pump** is another commonly used prosthetic device. This counterpulsation device usually is placed through the femoral artery and is synchronized with the cardiac cycle so that it expands in diastole, displacing its volume of blood, and collapses in systole, augmenting the cardiac output. A prominent "squishing" sound is heard in systole and diastole when an intraaortic balloon pump is used and may obscure normal heart sounds.

PERICARDIAL FRICTION RUB

A **pericardial friction rub** commonly is heard after coronary artery bypass graft (CABG) or cardiac valve surgery. This sound is loudest immediately after surgery and persists for several days and sometimes for 1 week.

A pericardial friction rub may recur weeks or months after surgery in patients experiencing postpericardiotomy syndrome. This syndrome mimics Dressler's syndrome, a postmyocardial infarction syndrome, and is believed to be an autoimmune reaction.

 Listen now to a patient with a pericardial friction rub. Refer to Chapter 11 for additional information on the pericardial friction rub.

The learner is advised to listen to cardiac surgery patients for pericardial friction rubs.

PACEMAKER SOUNDS

An endocardial pacemaker in the right ventricle gives an electrocardiogram (ECG) pattern of left bundle branch block. Therefore paradoxical splitting of the second heart sound (S_2) may be heard. This means that S_2 splits on expiration and becomes single on inspiration. This splitting is best heard at base left.

If the pacing wire should penetrate the myocardium, a pericardial friction rub may be heard. Occasionally a "clicking" sound just before the first heart sound also is heard in this situation because of stimulation of the intercostal or diaphragmatic muscle. The situation can be corrected by simply withdrawing the wire into the right ventricle.

A systolic murmur may be heard if tricuspid valve function is interrupted by the endocardial pacemaker when it is going through the valve. This murmur is best heard along the left lateral sternal border and is similar to that of tricuspid regurgitation.

Listen now to a paradoxical splitting of S$_2$ in a patient with an endocardial pacemaker in the right ventricle.

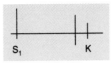

PERICARDIAL KNOCK

Pericardial knock, a sound occurring early in diastole after the second heart sound, is frequently heard in patients with constrictive pericarditis. This sound occurs slightly later than the opening snap of mitral stenosis but earlier than the third heart sound. This "knock" is a filling sound, with the pericardium acting as a constrictive membrane, preventing the usual relaxation of the ventricle in diastole.

Try to differentiate an opening snap from a pericardial knock or a left atrial myxoma "tumor plop."

 Listen now to a patient with a pericardial knock.

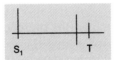

INTRACARDIAC MYXOMAS

A myxoma in the left atrium may mimic the heart sounds of mitral stenosis, except the louder-than-normal first heart sound is not present. A middiastolic rumble with a presystolic accentuation may be heard at the apex with the bell held lightly. An early diastolic sound resulting from the tumor striking the heart wall may be heard and is similar in timing to the opening snap of mitral stenosis. If the myxoma extends into the left ventricle, a systolic murmur similar to that of mitral regurgitation also may be heard. This latter murmur is best heard at the apex with the diaphragm pressed firmly.

 Listen now to a patient with a left atrial myxoma.

A myxoma in the right atrium produces a loud, early systolic sound usually regarded as a wide split first sound, which is best heard with the diaphragm at the left lateral sternal border. It also produces a pulmonic ejection murmur, which is best heard at base left. If the tumor extends into the right ventricle, a systolic murmur similar to that of tricuspid regurgitation also may be heard. This latter murmur is best heard at the left lateral sternal border, with the diaphragm firmly pressed.

Myxomas of the ventricles are rare. If they occur in the right ventricle, the murmur of pulmonic stenosis may be mimicked. A myxoma in the left ventricle would have an auscultatory murmur that mimics aortic stenosis.

STERNAL CLICK

After heart surgery requiring a median sternotomy, the sternum is assessed daily for signs of instability. One such sign is a sternal click, which is audible without a stethoscope when firm pressure is applied along the entire sternum with the fingertips. The presence of a click is indicative of sternal bone dehiscence, which is considered a warning sign of sternal infection. The click is thought to be produced by sternal-bone–to–sternal-bone motion. Having the patient cough while you apply sternal pressure will accentuate any instability.

SUBCUTANEOUS EMPHYSEMA

Subcutaneous emphysema, the presence of air or gas in the subcutaneous tissues, may be discerned with either palpation or auscultation. The area may appear puffy, and with slight pressure a "crackling" sound (crepitation) may be heard. The sound may be audible with or without the stethoscope over the area. It may occur when air escapes from a tracheostomy or thoracic incision and the air moves under the skin. The air may accumulate around the face, neck and throat, or thorax.

When subcutaneous emphysema occurs over the left chest, the crepitation should be recognized as a noncardiac sound. Generally, subcutaneous emphysema is not serious because the air is eventually reabsorbed by the body.

Its origin also may be a result of infection by gas-producing organisms, especially *Clostridium perfringens.* In the latter case, the puffiness and crepitation would appear in the area of the infection.

MEDIASTINAL CRUNCH

Mediastinal crunch is the presence of air in the mediastinum that produces a series of scratchy sounds, which correlate to either respiration or heartbeat but in a random fashion. The discovery of subcutaneous emphysema would confirm the presence of mediastinal crunch. These sounds commonly occur after cardiac surgery. A stethoscope usually is needed to hear them, although the patient may be aware of them.

SELF-LEARNING "UNKNOWN" HEART SOUNDS

 On the audio program, listen to the "unknown" heart sounds and identify the sound. Compare your answers with the answer key at the end of the chapter. Relisten to the audio program as needed to achieve mastery of the content.

1. Is the sound heard a pericardial friction rub, a paradoxical split second sound, a pericardial knock, or a left atrial myxoma?

2. Is the sound heard a left atrial myxoma, a pericardial friction rub, a pericardial knock, or a paradoxical split second sound?

3. Is the sound heard a paradoxical split second sound, a left atrial myxoma, a pericardial knock, or a pericardial friction rub?

4. Is the sound heard a pericardial friction rub, a paradoxical split second sound, a left atrial myxoma, or a pericardial knock?

SELF-LEARNING QUESTIONS

Select the letter of the correct response, or provide requested information. Compare your answers with the answer key at the end of the chapter. Reread the chapter as needed to achieve mastery of the content.

1. An endocardial pacemaker causes:
   a. physiological split of second sound
   b. paradoxical split of second sound
   c. split of first sound
   d. louder-than-normal first sound

2. The etiological factor of a pericardial knock is:
   a. constrictive pericarditis
   b. congestive heart failure
   c. uremic pericarditis
   d. none of the above

3. A sternal click is a sign of:
   a. mitral valve prolapse
   b. constrictive pericarditis
   c. unstable sternum
   d. subcutaneous emphysema

4. The sound heard when auscultating over subcutaneous emphysema is described as:
   a. crackling   b. click
   c. rub   d. scratchy

5. The sound heard when auscultating over the presence of air in the mediastinum is described as:
   a. crackling   b. click
   c. rub   d. scratchy

6. A myxoma in the left atrium has an early diastolic sound similar in timing to the opening snap but is from:
   a. mitral regurgitation   b. mitral stenosis
   c. tumor striking heart wall d. tumor extending into left ventricle

ANSWERS TO SELF-LEARNING "UNKNOWN" HEART SOUNDS

1. Pericardial friction rub

2. Paradoxical split second sound

3. Pericardial knock

4. Left atrial myxoma

ANSWERS TO SELF-LEARNING QUESTIONS

1. b

2. a

3. c

4. a

5. d

6. c

14

Common Adult Abnormalities

LEARNING OBJECTIVES

After reading this chapter, listening to the accompanying audio program, answering the self-learning questions at the end of the chapter, and listening to the "unknowns" on the audio program, the learner will be able to:

1. Identify common adult abnormalities with a systolic murmur.
2. Identify common adult abnormalities with a diastolic murmur.
3. Differentiate mitral regurgitation from aortic regurgitation.
4. Differentiate mitral stenosis from aortic stenosis.

When listening to adults, the clinician will encounter some common abnormalities. Every clinician should be able to differentiate these abnormalities from the normal heart. In this chapter a brief synopsis of the auscultatory findings in these abnormalities is given. The auscultatory findings use heart sounds that you learned in the previous chapters. If you have difficulty selectively listening to the sounds of the abnormality, you should review the previous chapters until you gain competency in the specific sound with which you are having difficulty. The real heart sounds used in this chapter are not added one by one as done previously. For complete assessment information on the abnormality, the clinician is advised to use other cardiac references that are readily available.

MITRAL REGURGITATION

Mitral regurgitation is the inability of the mitral valve to close completely, permitting backflow of blood from the left ventricle into the left atrium. It may be caused by either congenital or acquired disease. It is also known as *mitral incompetence* or *mitral insufficiency.*

The auscultatory findings of mitral regurgitation are:
1. Systolic murmur
    a. Late systolic (slight severity)
    b. Pansystolic (greater severity)
    c. Blowing quality
    d. High frequency
    e. Best heard with diaphragm chestpiece firmly pressed
    f. Best heard at apex
    g. Radiates toward left axilla or left lower sternal border; may radiate to base right (see Figure 7-1)
2. Wide split second sound (greater severity)
    a. High frequency
    b. Best heard with diaphragm chestpiece firmly pressed
    c. Best heard at base left
3. S_3 (if congestive heart failure [CHF] is also present)
    a. Low frequency
    b. Best heard with bell chestpiece lightly held
    c. Best heard at apex (left ventricular failure)

 Listen now to the sounds of mitral regurgitation as recorded from a real heart. You are listening at the apex with a bell chestpiece lightly held. Note the presence of an S_3.

TRICUSPID REGURGITATION

Tricuspid regurgitation is the inability of the tricuspid valve to close completely, permitting backflow of blood from the right ventricle into the right atrium. The disease is usually acquired; rheumatic fever is a common etiology. It is also known as *tricuspid incompetence* or *tricuspid insufficiency*. The auscultatory findings of tricuspid regurgitation are:

1. Systolic murmur
   a. Late systolic (slight severity)
   b. Pansystolic (greater severity)
   c. Blowing quality
   d. High frequency
   e. Best heard with diaphragm chestpiece firmly pressed
   f. Best heard at apex
   g. Radiates toward left axilla or left lower sternal border (see Figure 7-1)
2. Wide split second sound (greater severity)
   a. High frequency
   b. Best heard with diaphragm chestpiece firmly pressed
   c. Best heard at base left
3. S_3 (if CHF is also present)
   a. Low frequency
   b. Best heard with bell chestpiece lightly held
   c. Best heard at left lateral sternal border (LLSB) (right ventricular failure)
   d. Best heard at apex (left ventricular failure)

 Listen now to the sounds of tricuspid regurgitation as recorded from a real heart. You are listening at the LLSB with a diaphragm firmly pressed.

AORTIC STENOSIS

Aortic stenosis is the inability of the aortic valve to open completely, restricting blood flow from the left ventricle out into the aorta. A congenital bicuspid valve is often the etiology, but it may also be acquired. A narrow pulse pressure is a common physical finding, with a carotid pulse that is slow rising.

The auscultatory findings of aortic stenosis with moderate severity are:

1. Aortic ejection sound
   a. High frequency

    b. Best heard with diaphragm chestpiece firmly pressed

    c. Best heard at base right and on straight line from base right down to apex

  2. Systolic ejection murmur

    a. Harsh quality

    b. Medium frequency

    c. Heard equally well with either bell or diaphragm chestpiece

    d. Best heard at base right

    e. Radiates bilaterally into neck and down to apex (see Figure 7-1)

  3. Normal split S_1

  4. Physiological split S_2 (splits on inspiration; single on expiration)

    a. High frequency

    b. Best heard with diaphragm firmly pressed

    c. Heard at base right

The auscultatory findings of aortic stenosis with great severity are:

1. Aortic ejection sound absent

2. Systolic ejection murmur (grade III/VI or greater)

    a. Harsh quality

    b. Medium frequency

    c. Heard equally well with either bell or diaphragm chestpiece

    d. Best heard at base right

    e. Radiates bilaterally into neck and down to apex (see Figure 7-1)

3. Split S_1 may not be audible (M_1 closure muffled)

4. Physiological split S_2 may not be audible

5. S_4

    a. Low frequency

    b. Best heard with bell chestpiece lightly held

    c. Best heard at apex

 Listen now to the sounds of aortic stenosis as recorded from a real heart. An aortic ejection sound is heard and then the murmur of aortic stenosis. You are listening at base right.

PULMONIC STENOSIS

Pulmonic stenosis is the inability of the pulmonary valve to open completely, restricting blood flow from the right ventricle to the pulmonary artery. Its etiology is most commonly congenital, although it may be acquired. A narrow pulse pressure is found in this pathologic condition.

The auscultatory findings of pulmonic stenosis are:

1. Pulmonic ejection sound
   a. High frequency sound after S_1
   b. Best heard at base left and on a straight line from base left to the epigastric area
2. Systolic ejection murmur
   a. Harsh quality
   b. Medium frequency
   c. Heard equally well with either bell or diaphragm chestpiece
   d. Best heard at base left
   e. Radiates along upper left sternal border (see Figure 7-1)

 Listen now to the sounds of pulmonic stenosis as recorded from a real heart. A pulmonic ejection sound is first heard and then the murmur of pulmonic stenosis. You are listening at base left.

AORTIC REGURGITATION

Aortic regurgitation is the inability of the aortic valve to close completely, permitting backflow of blood from the aorta into the left ventricle. It may be caused by congenital or acquired disease. A wide pulse pressure is a common finding, with a rapid rising and collapsing pulse. It is also known as *aortic incompetence* or *aortic insufficiency.*

The auscultatory findings of aortic regurgitation are:

1. Aortic ejection sound (may not be present)
   a. High frequency
   b. Best heard with diaphragm chestpiece firmly pressed
   c. Best heard at base right and on straight line from base right down to apex
2. Early diastolic murmur
   a. Blowing quality
   b. High frequency
   c. Best heard with diaphragm chestpiece firmly pressed
   d. Best heard at Erb's point
   e. Radiates down lower left sternal border and to apex (see Figure 8-1)
   f. Having patient sit up and lean forward in deep exhalation or lean back on elbows brings out this soft murmur

 Listen now to the sounds of aortic regurgitation as recorded from a real heart. You are listening at Erb's point with a diaphragm firmly pressed and with the patient leaning forward.

PULMONIC REGURGITATION

Pulmonic regurgitation is the inability of the pulmonary valve to close completely, permitting backflow of blood from the pulmonary artery into the right ventricle. It is not a commonly acquired adult pathologic condition and is most often a congenital defect. A wide pulse pressure is a common finding.

The auscultatory findings of pulmonic regurgitation without pulmonary hypertension are:
1. Pulmonic ejection sound (may not be present)
   a. High frequency
   b. Best heard with diaphragm chestpiece firmly pressed
   c. Best heard at base left and on straight line from base left down to epigastrium
2. Early diastolic murmur
   a. Rough quality
   b. Mixed of low with some high frequencies
   c. Best heard with bell chestpiece lightly held
   d. Best heard at base left
   e. Radiates down upper left sternal border (see Figure 8-1)

 Listen now to the sounds of pulmonic regurgitation as recorded from a real heart. You are listening at base left with a diaphragm firmly pressed.

MITRAL STENOSIS

Mitral stenosis is the inability of the mitral valve to open completely, restricting blood flow from the left atrium to the left ventricle. Rheumatic fever is a common cause. Disease of the mitral valve is the most common worldwide valvular disease.

The auscultatory findings of mitral stenosis are:
1. Louder than normal S_1
   a. High frequency
   b. Best heard with diaphragm chestpiece firmly pressed
   c. Best heard at apex
2. Opening snap after S_2
   a. High frequency
   b. Best heard with diaphragm chestpiece firmly pressed
   c. Best heard at apex
3. Middiastolic ejection murmur
   a. Rumble quality

      b. Low frequency
      c. Best heard with bell chestpiece lightly held
      d. Best heard at apex
      e. Radiates to left axilla
   4. Late diastolic accentuation of murmur (also called *presystolic*)
      a. Rumble quality
      b. Low frequency
      c. Best heard with bell chestpiece lightly held
      d. Best heard at apex
      e. Radiates to left axilla (see Figure 8-1)

Listen now to the sounds of mitral stenosis as recorded from a real heart. You are listening at the apex with a bell chestpiece lightly held.

TRICUSPID STENOSIS

Tricuspid stenosis is the inability of the tricuspid valve to open completely, restricting blood flow from the right atrium to the right ventricle. Rheumatic fever is often the cause and therefore is frequently associated with mitral stenosis.

   The auscultatory findings of tricuspid stenosis are:
   1. Louder than normal S_1
      a. High frequency
      b. Best heard with diaphragm chestpiece firmly pressed
      c. Best heard at LLSB
   2. Opening snap after S_2
      a. High frequency
      b. Best heard with diaphragm chestpiece firmly pressed
      c. Best heard at LLSB
   3. Middiastolic ejection murmur
      a. Rumble quality
      b. Low frequency
      c. Best heard with bell chestpiece lightly held
      d. Best heard at LLSB
      e. Radiates down lower left sternal border
      f. Inspiration increases intensity of murmur
   4. Late diastolic accentuation of murmur (also called *presystolic*)
      a. Rumble quality
      b. Low frequency
      c. Best heard with bell chestpiece lightly held
      d. Best heard at LLSB

    e. Radiates down left sternal border (see Figure 8-1)

    f. Inspiration increases intensity of murmur

 Listen now to the sounds of tricuspid stenosis as recorded from a real heart. You are listening at left lateral sternal border with bell chestpiece lightly held.

SELF-LEARNING "UNKNOWN" HEART SOUNDS

 On the audio program, listen to the "unknown" heart sounds and identify the sound. Compare your answers with the answer key at the end of the chapter. Relisten to the audio program as needed to achieve mastery of the content.

You are listening at the apex with a diaphragm firmly pressed. The sound also radiates toward the left axilla and left sternal border. It may also radiate to base right. You hear the following sound.

  1. You identify the pathologic condition as:

    a. mitral stenosis   **b.** mitral regurgitation

    c. tricuspid stenosis   **d.** aortic stenosis

You are listening at base right with either a bell or diaphragm chestpiece. The sound also radiates bilaterally into the neck and down to the apex. You hear the following sound.

  2. You identify the pathologic condition as:

    a. mitral stenosis   **b.** mitral regurgitation

    c. tricuspid stenosis   **d.** aortic stenosis

SELF-LEARNING QUESTIONS

Select the letter of the correct response, or provide requested information. Compare your answers with the answer key at the end of the chapter. Reread the chapter as needed to achieve mastery of the content.

  1. List two common adult abnormalities that have a systolic murmur.

    a.

    b.

2. List two common adult abnormalities that have a diastolic murmur.
   a.
   b.

3. You are listening at the apex with a diaphragm firmly pressed and hear a loud first sound and an opening snap after the second sound. The pathologic condition you would suspect is:
   a. mitral regurgitation
   b. mitral stenosis
   c. aortic stenosis
   d. aortic regurgitation

ANSWERS TO SELF-LEARNING "UNKNOWN" HEART SOUNDS

1. b

2. d

ANSWERS TO SELF-LEARNING QUESTIONS

1. Any two of the following: mitral regurgitation, tricuspid regurgitation, aortic stenosis, pulmonic stenosis

2. Any two of the following: mitral stenosis, tricuspid stenosis, aortic regurgitation, pulmonic regurgitation

3. b

15

Geriatric Heart Sounds

LEARNING OBJECTIVES

After reading this chapter, listening to the accompanying audio program, answering the self-learning questions at the end of the chapter, and listening to the "unknowns" on the audio program, the learner will be able to do the following in the geriatric client:

1. List two auscultatory findings that change in the elderly.
2. By their heart sounds, differentiate aortic valve sclerosis from aortic valve stenosis.
3. Identify the most common condition causing a systolic murmur in the elderly.

GENERAL OBSERVATIONS

Accurate assessment of cardiac sounds may be more difficult in the elderly. This difficulty may be because of (1) increased anteroposterior chest diameter, especially at the base of the heart or (2) a very thin body structure, making it difficult to achieve a good air seal with the stethoscope. Also, some of the maneuvers used to differentiate pathologic conditions (e.g., squatting, the Valsalva) may not be feasible in the elderly.

HEART RATE

In the geriatric patient, a decreased resting heart rate with decreased cardiac output is not an infrequent occurrence. Heart rates as low as 40 beats/minute may be normal and may not adversely affect morbidity or mortality. This decreased heart rate and consequently decreased cardiac output are manifestations of decreased beta-adrenergic (vagal tone) responsiveness with aging. However, a normal slowing of the heart must be differentiated from an abnormal one caused by atrioventricular or intraventricular abnormal conduction.

SPLITTING OF FIRST AND SECOND SOUNDS

The splitting of S_1 is often more marked in the elderly and may be confused with an ejection sound or an S_4. The physiological split of the second sound may not be audible in the elderly as a result of prolongation of the left ventricular ejection and isovolumic contraction times.

S_4

The S_4 is seldom heard in younger adults except in well-conditioned athletes, but it may be heard in healthy older adults. Although common in the elderly, the S_4 is not necessarily normal and may be associated with heart disease. After age 75 years many have S_4 at the apex. They usually have left ventricular hypertrophy (LVH) and impaired diastolic relaxation on echocardiogram.

The auscultatory findings of an S_4 are:
1. Low-frequency sound in front of the first sound
2. Best heard at apex
3. Best heard with bell lightly held

S$_3$

An S$_3$ that is heard in anyone older than 40 years suggests either ventricular failure or volume overloading from valvular heart disease. Therefore an S$_3$ in older adults should not be considered physiological; it should be considered abnormal.

The auscultatory findings of pathological S$_3$ are:
1. Low-frequency sound after the second sound
2. Best heard at apex
3. Best heard with bell lightly held

AORTIC VALVE SCLEROSIS

Aortic valve sclerosis is the most common condition causing a systolic murmur in older adults. It may be found in up to 50% of those reaching 85 years. It results from degenerative fibrous thickening and stiffening of the base of the aortic cusps as they insert into the sinuses of Valsalva. This occurs without commissural fusion, without impairment of cusp mobility, and accordingly without obstruction. The condition may not be hemodynamically significant. Vascular stiffness found in the elderly may mask the narrow pulse pressure common in younger individuals.

The common auscultatory findings of aortic valve sclerosis are:
1. Systolic ejection murmur
   a. Murmur peaks early
   b. Harsh quality
   c. Heard equally well with either a bell or diaphragm chestpiece
   d. Best heard at base right
   e. Rarely radiates to the carotid arteries
   f. May be considered an "innocent" murmur

 Listen now to the sounds of aortic sclerosis as recorded from a real heart. You are listening at base right with either a bell or diaphragm chestpiece.

AORTIC VALVE STENOSIS

Aortic stenosis increases with age. A congenitally abnormal aortic valve may manifest calcific degeneration in the sixth decade of life, whereas a previously normal aortic valve may not manifest such changes until the seventh decade. The classic narrow pulse pressure found in younger adults with aortic stenosis may be absent in the elderly. The carotid upstroke may not be slow in the elderly as it is in younger adults, because vascular compliance is diminished.

The auscultatory findings of aortic valve stenosis with **moderate** stenosis are:

1. Systolic ejection murmur
   a. Murmur less intense in the elderly
   b. Harsh quality
   c. Heard equally well with either bell or diaphragm
   d. Best heard at base right
   e. Radiates down to apex and bilaterally into neck (see Figure 7-1)
2. Aortic ejection sound
   a. Usually not audible in the elderly
   b. If present, high frequency
   c. Best heard with diaphragm
   d. Best heard at base right and on straight line down to apex
3. Normal split S_1
   a. Heard at fourth intercostal space (ICS) at left sternal border
   b. Heard with diaphragm
   c. May be increased and confused with ejection sound or S_4
4. Physiological split S_2 (splits on inspiration; single on expiration)
   a. May not be audible in the elderly
   b. Heard at base right
   c. Best heard with diaphragm

The auscultatory findings of aortic valve stenosis with **severe** stenosis are:

1. Systolic ejection murmur
   a. May be less than grade II/VI in intensity
   b. Harsh quality
   c. Heard equally well with either bell or diaphragm
   d. Best heard at base right
   e. Radiates down to apex and bilaterally into neck
2. M_1 closure muffled (split S_1 not heard at left lateral sternal border [LLSB])
3. Aortic ejection sound absent
4. S_4
   a. Low-frequency sound in front of S_1
   b. Best heard at apex
   c. Heard with bell lightly held

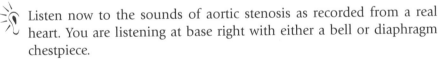 Listen now to the sounds of aortic stenosis as recorded from a real heart. You are listening at base right with either a bell or diaphragm chestpiece.

MITRAL REGURGITATION

The aging process may affect the mitral valve, usually about a decade after it affects the aortic valve. The degenerative changes with calcification of the mitral annulus or valve ring hinder the normal contraction of the ring during systole. This produces a systolic murmur of **mitral regurgitation**.

The auscultatory findings of mitral regurgitation are:
1. Systolic murmur
   a. Late systolic (slight regurgitation)
   b. Holosystolic (severe regurgitation)
   c. Blowing quality
   d. Best heard with diaphragm
   e. Best heard at apex
   f. Radiates to left axilla and left sternal border; may radiate to base left (see Figure 7-1)
2. Wide split second
   a. May not be audible in the elderly
   b. If audible, heard at base right
   c. Heard with diaphragm
3. S_3
   a. Low frequency sound after S_2
   b. Best heard at apex
   c. Heard with bell lightly held

 Listen now to the sounds of mitral regurgitation as recorded from a real heart. You are listening at the apex with a diaphragm chestpiece firmly pressed. Note the presence of an S_3.

TRICUSPID REGURGITATION

Pure **tricuspid regurgitation** is uncommon in the elderly but may be a component of pulmonary hypertension. With pulmonary hypertension, the right ventricle dilates, which stretches the tricuspid annulus, and the valve therefore becomes incompetent.

The auscultatory findings of tricuspid regurgitation are:
1. Systolic murmur
   a. Late systolic (slight regurgitation)
   b. Holosystolic (severe regurgitation)
   c. Blowing quality
   d. Best heard with diaphragm
   e. Best heard at apex
   f. Radiates to left axilla and left sternal border (see Figure 7-1.)

2. Wide split second
    a. May not be audible in the elderly
    b. If audible, heard at base right
    c. Heard with diaphragm
3. S_3
    a. Low-frequency sound after S_2
    b. Best heard at apex
    c. Heard with bell lightly held

 Listen now to the sounds of tricuspid regurgitation as recorded from a real heart. You are listening at left sternal border with a diaphragm chestpiece firmly pressed.

DIASTOLIC MURMURS

Diastolic murmurs are considered pathological at any age. Pathological conditions generating diastolic murmurs include mitral or tricuspid stenosis and aortic or pulmonic regurgitation.

MITRAL STENOSIS

In the elderly **mitral stenosis**, which is usually of rheumatic origin, may not become acutely symptomatic except if atrial fibrillation suddenly develops.

The auscultatory findings of mitral stenosis are:
1. Louder than normal first sound
    a. Best heard at LLSB
    b. Best heard with diaphragm
2. Opening snap after second sound
    a. Heard at apex
    b. Best heard with diaphragm
3. Middiastolic murmur
    a. Rumble quality
    b. Best heard with bell lightly held
    c. Best heard at apex
    d. Radiates to left axilla (see Figure 8-1)

 Listen now to the sounds of mitral stenosis as recorded from a real heart. You are listening at the apex with a bell chestpiece lightly held.

TRICUSPID STENOSIS

In the elderly **tricuspid stenosis** is rare and is seen most often in multivalvular rheumatic disease. Patients with isolated tricuspid stenosis will manifest signs of right heart failure.

The auscultatory findings of pure tricuspid stenosis are:
1. Louder than normal first sound
   a. Best heard at LLSB
   b. Best heard with diaphragm
2. Opening snap after second sound
   a. Heard at LLSB
   b. Best heard with diaphragm
3. Middiastolic murmur
   a. Rumble quality
   b. Best heard with bell lightly held
   c. Best heard at LLSB
   d. Radiates along left sternal border
   e. Inspiration increases intensity of murmur (see Figure 8-1)

 Listen now to the sounds of tricuspid stenosis as recorded from a real heart. You are listening at the left sternal border with a diaphragm chestpiece firmly pressed.

AORTIC REGURGITATION

Aortic regurgitation is less common in the elderly than is aortic stenosis. It may be caused by valvular degeneration, congenital bicuspid aortic valve, rheumatic heart disease, infective endocarditis, or systemic arterial hypertension.

The auscultatory findings of aortic regurgitation are:
1. Early diastolic murmur
   a. Blowing quality
   b. Best heard at Erb's point
   c. Best heard with diaphragm
   d. Radiates down left sternal border (see Figure 8-1)
   e. Having patient sit up and lean forward in deep exhalation or lean back on elbows brings out this soft murmur
2. Aortic ejection sound after S_1
   a. Usually not audible in the elderly
   b. If present, high frequency
   c. Best heard with diaphragm
   d. Best heard at base right and on straight line down to apex

Listen now to the sounds of aortic regurgitation as recorded from a real heart. You are listening at Erb's point with a diaphragm chestpiece firmly pressed. The patient is leaning forward.

PULMONIC REGURGITATION

In the elderly, **pulmonic regurgitation** is usually a result of pulmonary hypertension that is caused by left-sided heart failure or primary pulmonary disease.

The auscultatory findings of pulmonic regurgitation are:
1. Early diastolic murmur
    a. Rough quality
    b. Best heard at base left
    c. Best heard with bell
    d. Radiates along upper left sternal border (see Figure 8-1)
2. Pulmonic ejection sound (may not be present)
    a. High-frequency sound after S_1
    b. Best heard at base left and on straight line down to epigastrium

 Listen now to the sounds of pulmonic regurgitation as recorded from a real heart. You are listening at base left with a diaphragm chestpiece firmly pressed.

SELF-LEARNING "UNKNOWN" HEART SOUNDS

 On the audio program, listen to the "unknown" heart sounds and identify the sound. Compare your answers with the answer key at the end of the chapter. Relisten to the audio program as needed to achieve mastery of the content.

You are listening at the apex with a diaphragm firmly pressed. The sound also radiates toward the left axilla and left sternal border. It may also radiate to base right. You hear the following sound.

1. You identify the pathologic condition as:
    a. mitral stenosis
    b. mitral regurgitation
    c. tricuspid stenosis
    d. aortic stenosis

You are listening at base right with either a bell or diaphragm chestpiece.

The sound also radiates bilaterally into the neck and down to the apex. You hear the following sound.

2. You identify the pathologic condition as:
   a. mitral stenosis
   b. mitral regurgitation
   c. aortic stenosis
   d. tricuspid stenosis

SELF-LEARNING QUESTIONS

Select the letter of the correct response, or provide requested information. Compare your answers with the answer key at the end of the chapter. Reread the chapter as needed to achieve mastery of the content.

1. List two auscultatory findings that change in the elderly.
   a.
   b.

2. The systolic ejection murmur that is best heard at base right and radiates bilaterally into the neck and down to the apex is that of:
   a. aortic sclerosis
   b. aortic stenosis
   c. aortic regurgitation
   d. none of the above

ANSWERS TO SELF-LEARNING "UNKNOWN" HEART SOUNDS

1. b

2. c

ANSWERS TO SELF-LEARNING QUESTIONS

1. Any two of the following: heart rate decreased, cardiac output decreased, splitting of S_1 more marked, physiological S_4, pathological S_3

2. b

16

Introduction to Pediatric Auscultation

LEARNING OBJECTIVES

After reading this chapter, listening to the accompanying audio program, answering the self-learning questions at the end of the chapter, and listening to the "unknowns" on the audio program, the learner will be able to do the following in infants and children:

1. Identify changing position of the point of maximum impulse (PMI) with advancing age.
2. Identify heart rate appropriate for different ages.
3. Identify areas to auscultate.
4. Identify physiological split second sound.
5. Differentiate S_3 from S_4.
6. Differentiate split second from S_3 or S_4.

FETAL HEART SOUNDS

The sounds from the **fetal heart** heard through the maternal abdomen in pregnancy are known as *fetal heart sounds*. Until the mid-1960s, the fetal heartbeat was listened to through various stethoscopes including a head stethoscope (the fetoscope). Today the fetal heartbeat is monitored most frequently using an electronic monitoring device. The fetal heart is monitored during pregnancy, and monitoring is especially helpful during labor. The goal of monitoring, either by auscultation or electronic means, is to detect fetal stress or distress so that appropriate interventions can be taken to alleviate its cause.

PEDIATRIC AUSCULTATION

Auscultation is the core of the pediatric cardiovascular evaluation, but listening to the pediatric heart has more challenges than listening to the adult heart. You must first complete the auscultation without producing a physical struggle or a crying or distraught patient. For infants, you may wish to do as much of the assessment in the parent's arms if this helps to keep the infant content and quiet. Auscultate before performing disturbing or uncomfortable aspects of the physical assessment. Toddlers prefer to make the first move, and allowing them to play with an old stethoscope while you take the history from the parent may facilitate the toddler's cooperation. School-age children like to know what you are going to do and what you expect from them. Tell them this when you meet and as you proceed through the examination. Once you have mastered keeping the infant or child quiet and content, you will find that many of the sounds you learned for an adult are comparable in pediatric patients. Therefore, if you know how to listen and interpret adult heart sounds, you have only a few things to learn to listen to the pediatric heart. Some of the differences include the areas to auscultate, location of the apical impulse, the heart rate, and pathologic conditions specific to the infant or child.

AREAS TO AUSCULTATE

The normal **auscultatory areas** that you learned in Chapter 1 are applicable for the infant and child (Figure 16-1). In addition to the areas over the anterior chest, it may be helpful to listen to three areas on the back: (1) left atrial area, (2) aortic area, and (3) pulmonic area. See Table 16-1 for the location of these posterior areas and the murmurs commonly radiating to the areas.

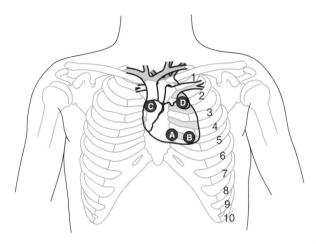

Figure 16-1   Sites for auscultation in infant or child. **A,** Left lateral sternal border (sounds from tricuspid valve and right side of heart best heard); **B,** apex (sounds from mitral valve and left side of heart best heard); **C,** base right (sounds from aortic valve best heard); **D,** base left (sounds from pulmonic valve best heard).

TABLE 16-1
Posterior Auscultatory Areas

Area Name	Location	Murmur Radiating to Area
Left atrial	5th-8th Left posterior interspaces	Mitral regurgitation
Aortic	4th-8th Thoracic vertebral bodies to left of midline	Aortic stenosis Aortic regurgitation
Pulmonic	4th-5th Thoracic vertebrae, left and right of spine	Pulmonic stenosis Pulmonic regurgitation Atrial septal defect

It is important to keep in mind that in pediatric auscultation, congenital malformations may cause the heart, blood vessels, or valves to be in an abnormal location. Therefore, listen to all areas with a bell and diaphragm and then describe where an abnormality is best heard and where it radiates.

APICAL IMPULSE

The **apical impulse** (point of maximal impulse [PMI]) is at the level of the fourth intercostal space (ICS) until age 7 years, when it drops to the fifth ICS. This impulse is also often visible in infants and young children. It is

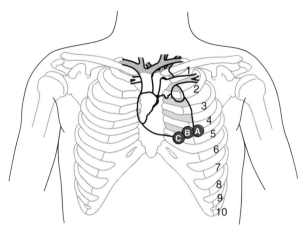

Figure 16-2   Point of maximal impulse (PMI). **A,** Site until age 4 years; **B,** site ages 4-6 years; **C,** site ages 7 years and older.

to the left of the midclavicular line until age 4 years, is at the midclavicular line between ages 4 and 6 years, and moves to the right at age 7 years (Figure 16-2).

HEART RATE

Fetal

The normal range for the **fetal heart rate** is 120 to 160 beats/minute (Table 16-2). The rate varies with the fetus' behavioral/waking status. However, a rate over 160 beats/ minute for more than 10 consecutive minutes may be indicative of maternal fever or anxiety, fetal anemia or tachyarrhythmia, or dehydration. A decrease in rate to below 120 beats/minute for 10 consecutive minutes may result from medications or hypoxia. Definitions vary for fetal heart rate abnormalities and the criteria for interventions resulting from fetal heart monitoring. These definitions and interventions are based largely on experience and expert opinion. It is not the purpose of this book to discuss fetal monitoring in any detail but merely to mention its existence. Clinicians needing expertise in this specialty should refer to other sources that cover it.

 Listen now to a fetal heart rate of 130 beats/minute. You are listening over the pregnant abdomen with a fetoscope.

Newborn

The normal **newborn's** heart rate is between 70 and 120 beats/minute, but with activity such as crying, stress, or fever, it may increase to 220

TABLE 16-2
Advancing Age and Normal Heart Rates at Rest in Beats/Minute

Age	Lower Limits	Average	Upper Limits
Fetal	120	140	160
Newborn	70	120	170
1-12 months	80	120	160
1-7 years	75	100	130
8-17 years	70	90	110
18 years or older	50	75	95

beats/minute. The heart rate normally will decrease during sleep and/or vagal stimulation. A heart rate consistently over 170 in an infant or over 130 in a toddler, not explained by activity, stress, or fever, should be considered abnormal. As the infant advances in age, the heart rate decreases (see Table 16-2).

 Listen now to a newborn with a heart rate of 130 beats/minute. You are listening at the apex with a diaphragm chestpiece firmly pressed.

S_3

The concepts learned in Chapter 5 regarding the S_3 are applicable to infants and children. As indicated earlier, an S_3 is normal in children and young adults because of the increased diastolic volumes that are usually present. However, this "normal," or nonpathological, S_3 is usually absent by the time males reach their late 20s and females their 30s.

An S_3 of left ventricular origin is best heard at the PMI, which changes with advancing age (see Figure 16-2). An S_3 of right ventricular origin is loudest from birth to age 6 years at the fourth intercostal space along the left lateral sternal border (LLSB). At age 7 years, it is best heard at the fifth intercostal space at LLSB.

Although an S_3 heard in an infant or child may be normal, it may also be indicative of underlying heart failure or a large left-to-right shunt. The pathological S_3 is usually palpable, whereas the physiological S_3 is not. Because the S_3 is a low frequency sound, it is best heard with a bell lightly held over the PMI as appropriate for the age of the child being auscultated.

 Listen now to an S_3 at a heart rate of 130 beats/minute. You are listening at the apex with a bell chestpiece lightly held.

S$_4$

The S$_4$ is not usually a normal finding in an infant or a child, although it may be normal in a young person who is an energetically trained athlete. More often than not, an S$_4$ that is heard in an infant or child is abnormal. However, the concepts learned in Chapter 4 regarding the S$_4$ are also applicable here.

The S$_4$ may be of either right or left ventricular origin. Those of right ventricular origin are most common and are best heard from birth to age 6 years at the fourth intercostal space along the LLSB. At age 7 years, it is best heard at the fifth intercostal space at LLSB. Common pathologic conditions having an S$_4$ of right ventricular origin are (1) primary pulmonary hypertension, (2) pulmonic stenosis, (3) Ebstein's anomaly, (4) tricuspid atresia, (5) total anomalous pulmonary venous return, and (6) complete heart block. An S$_4$ of left ventricular origin is best heard at the PMI (see Figure 16-2). Common pathologic conditions having an S$_4$ of left ventricular origin are (1) severe left ventricular disease, (2) aortic stenosis, and (3) coarctation of the aorta.

 Listen now to an S$_4$. You are listening at the apex with a bell chestpiece lightly held.

QUADRUPLE RHYTHM

In a vigorously trained athlete child, both a normal S$_3$ and S$_4$ may be audible and is known as a *quadruple rhythm*. In this rhythm the S$_4$, S$_1$, S$_2$, and S$_3$ are distinctly audible. As low frequency sounds, the S$_4$ and S$_3$ are heard with the bell chestpiece lightly held. The higher frequency sounds of S$_1$ and S$_2$ are best heard with the diaphragm chestpiece firmly pressed. This quadruple rhythm is best heard at the apex.

 Listen now to a quadruple rhythm. You are listening at the apex with a bell chestpiece lightly held.

SUMMATION GALLOP

When both S$_3$ and S$_4$ are present, especially at a rapid rate, they may be perceived as a single sound that is known as a *summation gallop*. It is the most common "gallop" heard in the infant or child and is usually a sign of congestive heart failure. This fusion of the S$_3$ and S$_4$ occurs because the tachycardia shortens diastole. The gallop is best heard at the apex with a bell lightly held.

Listen now to a summation gallop. You are listening at the apex with a bell chestpiece lightly held.

SPLIT SECOND SOUND

Physiological Split

Normally **the physiological split** S$_2$, a second sound that splits on inspiration and becomes single on expiration, is heard in infants and children. However, this normal splitting of the second sound is not heard in newborns until after the high resistance in the pulmonary circulation that is normal in fetal life falls. This pulmonary circulation resistance initially falls dramatically at birth but does not reach levels considered normal until the infant is 6 to 8 weeks old. After this time, a physiological split becomes audible. See Chapter 3 for further information regarding the physiological split second. In assessing the hearts of infants or children, the presence or absence of the physiologic split is important diagnostically and should always be determined. The split second is best heard at base left, second interspace to the left of the sternum, with the diaphragm firmly pressed.

 Listen now to a physiological split second. Note that the split is heard during inspiration and is not heard during expiration. You are listening at base left with a diaphragm firmly pressed.

Fixed Split

Fixed splitting of S$_2$, in which the split does not change during inspiration or expiration, is a diagnostic sign of atrial septal defect. See Chapter 10 for further discussion on the fixed split S$_2$.

 Listen now to a fixed split S$_2$. You are listening at base left with a diaphragm firmly pressed.

SELF-LEARNING "UNKNOWN" HEART SOUNDS

 On the audio program, listen to the "unknown" heart sounds and identify the sound. Compare your answers with the answer key at the end of the chapter. Relisten to the audio program as needed to achieve mastery of the content.

You are listening to the heart at base left with the diaphragm applied firmly.

1. The S_2 split is:
   a. physiological
   b. fixed split

You are listening to the heart at base left with the diaphragm applied firmly.

2. The S_2 split is:
   a. physiological
   b. fixed split

You are listening to the heart at the apex with a bell chestpiece lightly held.

3. You hear an:
   a. S_4
   b. S_3

SELF-LEARNING QUESTIONS

Select the letter of the correct response. Compare your answers with the answer key at the end of the chapter. Reread the chapter as needed to achieve mastery of the content.

1. The normal heart rate in beats/minute for a child of age 2 years is:
   a. 75-130   b. 120-160
   c. 50-95   d. 70-110

2. The point of maximal impulse (PMI) for a normal 5-year-old is at the:
   a. fifth ICS at midclavicular line
   b. fourth ICS at midclavicular line
   c. fifth ICS and left of midclavicular line
   d. fourth ICS and left of midclavicular line

3. A split of S_2 that does not change its width with inspiration or expiration is descriptive of a:
   a. physiological split S_2 b. paradoxical split S_2
   c. fixed split S_2 d. narrow split S_2

4. An S_3 that is physiological may be heard in a female until age:
   a. 5 years   b. 10 years
   c. 20 years   d. 30 years

5. An S_4 in a child is considered:
   a. abnormal
   c. normal

   b. a sign of congestive heart failure
   d. a sign of high pulmonary pressure

ANSWERS TO SELF-LEARNING "UNKNOWN" HEART SOUNDS

1. a

2. b

3. b

ANSWERS TO SELF-LEARNING QUESTIONS

1. a

2. b

3. c

4. d

5. a

Pediatric Systolic Murmurs

LEARNING OBJECTIVES

After reading this chapter, listening to the accompanying audio program, answering the self-learning questions at the end of the chapter, and listening to the "unknowns" on the audio program, the learner will be able to do the following in infants and children:

1. Identify two of the physical findings common to those with an innocent murmur.
2. Recognize the most common innocent murmur.
3. Recognize the name given to any condition having a left-to-right shunt that reverses to become a right-to-left shunt.
4. Identify the most common pathologic condition that causes a systolic murmur in a child.

INNOCENT MURMURS

An **innocent murmur** is a benign or functional continuous sound that is caused by a normal degree of turbulence as blood moves from one area to another. This turbulence sets the surrounding tissues into vibration, which is transmitted out through the chest and to the stethoscope. Innocent murmurs are ejection in type and a grade I or II in intensity without any other sign or symptom of heart disease. It is important to remember that a physiological split S_2 is also present in these children. These murmurs do not require follow-up care, nor do they need to be evaluated by a pediatric cardiologist. It is estimated that an innocent, or benign, systolic murmur may be audible in up to 90% of children. Therefore it is important that innocent murmurs be identified and differentiated from pathological murmurs.

The physical findings common to those with innocent or benign murmurs are:
1. Precordial activity is normal.
2. First heart sound is normal.
3. Second heart sound splits physiologically (splits on inspiration and becomes single on expiration).
4. Systolic murmur decreases in intensity on standing. (Most pathological murmurs do not change significantly with standing. The exception is the murmur of hypertrophic obstructive cardiomyopathy [HOCM]. The murmur of this condition increases in intensity when the person stands. Although the condition is rare, it is one of the leading causes of sudden death in athletes.)

Six murmurs may be considered innocent and include (1) Still's murmur, (2) physiologic systolic ejection murmur, (3) arterial supraclavicular bruit, (4) pulmonary flow murmur, (5) cervical venous hum, and (6) mammary soufflé.

STILL'S MURMUR

This is the most common innocent or normal murmur. It was first described by Dr. Still in 1909. It is thought to originate from periodic vibrations of the pulmonic leaflets at their attachments.

The auscultatory findings of a Still's murmur include:
1. Early systolic to midsystolic murmur
   a. Medium frequency
   b. Groaning, twanging quality
   c. Equally well heard with either the bell or the diaphragm chestpiece

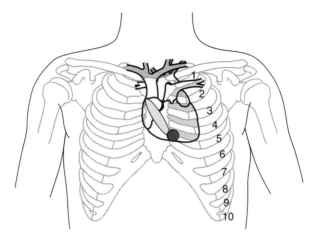

Figure 17-1   Still's murmur. *Circled* area site best heard. *Shaded* area indicates radiation.

      d. Best heard over the right ventricle between the left lateral sternal border (LLSB) and the apexe. Radiates toward base right (Figure 17-1)
      f. Murmur is decreased by standing or the Valsalva maneuver
   2. Differential diagnoses include aortic stenosis, HOCM, or a small ventricular septal defect (VSD)

 Listen now to Still's murmur from a real heart. You are listening over the right ventricle between the LLSB and the apex with either the bell or diaphragm chestpiece.

PHYSIOLOGIC SYSTOLIC EJECTION MURMUR

A common innocent murmur is caused by flow of blood as it is ejected from the left ventricle.

    The auscultatory findings of a physiologic systolic ejection murmur are:
   1. Systolic ejection murmur
      a. High frequency
      b. Blowing quality
      c. Best heard with diaphragm firmly pressed
      d. Best heard at left midsternal to upper sternal border
   2. Physiological split second sound (splits on inspiration; single on expiration)
      a. High frequency
      b. Best heard with diaphragm firmly pressed
      c. Heard at base left (Figure 17-2)

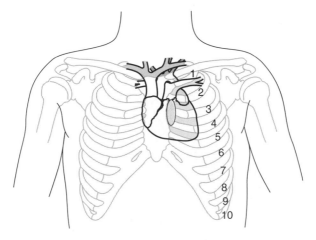

Figure 17-2   Physiologic systolic ejection murmur. *Shaded* area where heard.

3. This is the type of murmur that is also heard during pregnancy.

 Listen now to a physiologic systolic ejection murmur from a real heart. You are listening over the left midsternal to upper sternal border with a diaphragm chestpiece firmly pressed.

ARTERIAL SUPRACLAVICULAR BRUIT

Another innocent murmur is the **arterial supraclavicular bruit**. It is attributed to turbulence at the origins of the brachiocephalic vessels.

The auscultatory findings of arterial supraclavicular bruit include:
1. Brief early systolic ejection bruit
    a. Low frequency
    b. Best heard with bell lightly held
    c. Best heard in supraclavicular fossa; above and not below clavicle; right side greater than left (Figure 17-3)
    d. May also be audible in lower neck but does not radiate
    e. Reduced or vanishes with shoulder hyperextension
2. No ejection sound

PULMONARY FLOW MURMUR

Of all innocent murmurs of childhood, especially in newborn or premature infants, 15% are related to an innocent **pulmonary flow murmur**. This murmur results from turbulence caused by changes in

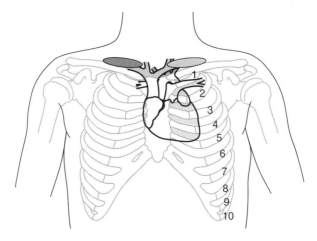

Figure 17-3   Arterial supraclavicular bruit. *Shaded* area indicates where heard.

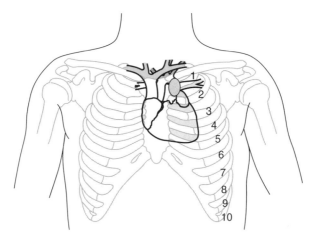

Figure 17-4   Innocent pulmonary flow murmur. *Shaded* area indicates where heard.

systolic pressure from the pulmonary trunk to its branches. It disappears, usually within a few months, as the infant grows.

The auscultatory findings of a pulmonary flow murmur include:

1. Midsystolic murmur
   a. Grade I-II
   b. Medium pitched
   c. Heard equally well with either bell or diaphragm chestpiece
   d. Maximal at base left (Figure 17-4)
   e. Does not radiate to back or neck
   f. Increased in high-output states such as anemia, thyrotoxicosis

2. No ejection sound heard
3. Physiologic split S_2 (splits on inspiration; single on expiration)
   a. High frequency
   b. Best heard with diaphragm firmly pressed
   c. Best heard at base left
4. Its differential diagnoses are atrial septal defect (ASD), pulmonic stenosis, tricuspid regurgitation, and HOCM

 Listen now to a pulmonary flow murmur from a real heart. You are listening over base left with either the bell or diaphragm chestpiece.

CERVICAL VENOUS HUM

This is the second most common innocent murmur of toddlers to school-age children. Because this murmur has both a systolic and diastolic component, it is discussed in Chapter 19.

MAMMARY SOUFFLÉ

The **mammary soufflé** is an innocent murmur that may be heard in the latter months of pregnancy or during lactation. Because this murmur may have both a systolic and diastolic component, it is discussed in Chapter 19.

MITRAL VALVE PROLAPSE

As with adults, the diagnosis of **mitral valve prolapse** should be made on auscultatory findings that are then confirmed by an echocardiogram. See Chapter 9 for additional information on mitral valve prolapse.

The auscultatory findings of mitral valve prolapse include:
1. Midsystolic click (may be the only auscultatory feature in a child)
   a. High frequency sound after S_1
   b. Best heard with diaphragm
   c. Best heard at apex or toward LLSB (Figure 17-5)
   d. Click accentuated on having child stand; may be inaudible when child is lying
2. Late systolic murmur (if mitral leaflets separate and permit regurgitation of blood from left ventricle into left atrium; not common in children)
   a. High frequency blow (also described as *honk* or *whoop*)

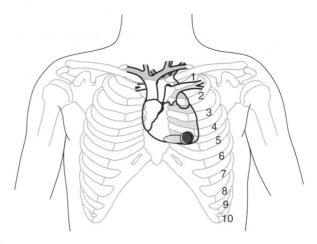

Figure 17-5   Mitral valve prolapse. *Circled* area site best heard. *Shaded* area indicates radiation.

b. Best heard with diaphragm
c. Best heard at apex or toward left sternal border

 Listen now to mitral valve prolapse from a real heart. You are listening at the apex with a diaphragm chestpiece firmly pressed.

MITRAL REGURGITATION

Mitral regurgitation in children is associated with either congenital or acquired pathologic conditions. Congenital causes may include endocardial cushion defects or mitral valve prolapse. Acquired disease may result from rheumatic fever or after correction of an atrial septal defect.

The auscultatory findings of mitral regurgitation are:
1. Systolic murmur
   a. Late systolic (slight severity)
   b. Pansystolic (severe)
   c. Blowing quality
   d. Best heard with diaphragm
   e. Best heard at apex
   f. Radiates to left axilla and LLSB. May radiate to back between left fifth and eighth intercostal spaces (ICS) (Figure 17-6)
2. Wide split second sound
   a. High frequency
   b. Best heard with diaphragm
   c. Heard at base left

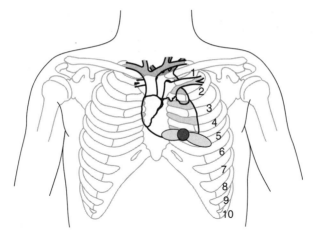

Figure 17-6   Mitral regurgitation. *Circled* area site best heard. *Shaded* area indicates radiation.

3. S$_3$
   a. Low frequency sound after S$_2$
   b. Best heard with bell lightly held
   c. Heard at apex

 Listen now to mitral regurgitation from a real heart. You are listening at the apex with a bell chestpiece lightly held. Note the audible S$_3$. If pressure were put on the bell, the S$_3$ would diminish or go away and the murmur would be more audible. (This feature is not demonstrated.)

TRICUSPID REGURGITATION

Tricuspid regurgitation in children may be the result of a large ventricular septal defect with pulmonary hypertension, rheumatic fever, or surgical repairs of complete transposition of the great arteries or tetralogy of Fallot.

The auscultatory findings of tricuspid regurgitation are:
1. Systolic murmur
   a. Late systolic (slight severity)
   b. Pansystolic (severe)
   c. Blowing quality
   d. Best heard with diaphragm
   e. Best heard at LLSB (Figure 17-7)
   f. Radiates down left sternal border
   g. Murmur loudest during inspiration and softer during expiration

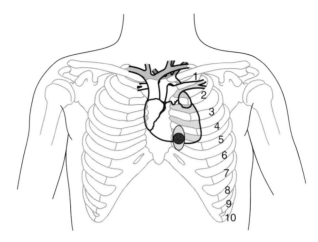

Figure 17-7   Tricuspid regurgitation. *Circled* area site best heard. *Shaded* area indicates radiation.

2. P₂ component increased
   a. High frequency sound
   b. Best heard with diaphragm
   c. Heard at base left
3. S₃
   a. Low frequency sound after S₂
   b. Best heard with bell lightly held
   c. Heard at apex

 Listen now to tricuspid regurgitation from a real heart. You are listening at the apex with a diaphragm chestpiece firmly pressed.

AORTIC VALVE STENOSIS

Congenital **aortic valve stenosis** is usually caused by malformed cusps resulting in a bicuspid valve, although obstruction to flow from the left ventricle to the aorta may be located below the aortic valve (subvalvular), at the aortic valve (valvular), or just above the valve (supravalvular). With any of these obstructions, left ventricular pressure must be increased to maintain normal aortic flow. This increased pressure leads to left ventricular hypertrophy, dilation, and cardiac failure. A thrill is usually palpable over the left ventricle.

The auscultatory findings of aortic stenosis include:
1. Systolic ejection murmur
   a. Mix of high and low frequencies

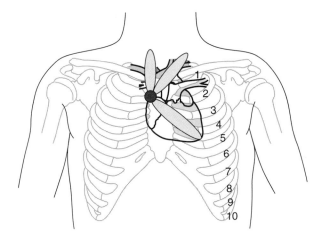

Figure 17-8   Aortic valve stenosis. *Circled* area site best heard. *Shaded* area indicates radiation.

    b. Harsh quality
    c. Equally well heard with either bell or diaphragm chestpiece
    d. Best heard at base right (in children younger than 5 years, may be loudest at left sternal border and toward apex) (Figure 17-8)
    e. Radiates bilaterally into neck and down to apex. May radiate to back between fourth and eighth thoracic vertebral bodies to left of midline
    f. Murmur becomes louder and longer and peaks later with increased severity
  2. Aortic ejection sound (present in valvular stenosis; absent in subvalvular stenosis [in aortic ring])
    a. High frequency sound
    b. Best heard with diaphragm
    c. Heard on straight line from base right to apex
  3. Narrow split second (A_2 component may be delayed)
    a. High-frequency sound
    b. Best heard with diaphragm
    c. Heard at base left
  4. S_3 (pathological if child is in congestive heart failure [CHF]; sounds same as physiological S_3)
    a. Low frequency sound after S_2
    b. Best heard with bell lightly held
    c. Best heard at apex

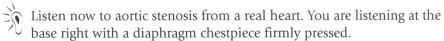 Listen now to aortic stenosis from a real heart. You are listening at the base right with a diaphragm chestpiece firmly pressed.

PULMONIC VALVE STENOSIS

In the child the etiology of **pulmonic valve stenosis** is congenitally altered or distorted pulmonary valve cusps that during development fuse and form a membrane with a small opening in the center. Because the lesion obstructs the flow of blood from the right ventricle, the level of right ventricular pressure must increase to maintain a normal blood flow into the pulmonary artery. With this high pressure, enlargement of the right ventricle and occasionally the right atrium occurs. About one third of children with this lesion will also have an atrial septal defect (ASD). For sounds heard in ASD, see Chapter 19.

The auscultatory findings in children with only a pulmonic valve stenosis are:

1. Systolic ejection murmur
   a. Mix of high and low frequencies
   b. Harsh quality
   c. Equally well heard with either bell or diaphragm chestpiece
   d. Best heard at base left (Figure 17-9)
   e. Radiates to suprasternal notch and along left sternal border; may radiate to back between fourth and eighth thoracic vertebral bodies to left of midline
2. Wide split second sound (varies with respiration; wide on expiration but wider still on inspiration)
   a. High frequency sound
   b. Best heard with diaphragm chestpiece
   c. Best heard at base left
   d. The tighter the pulmonic stenosis, the wider the split

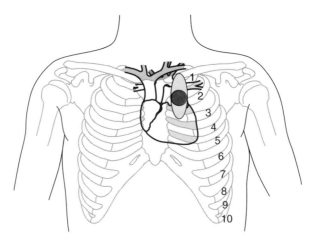

Figure 17-9   Pulmonic valve stenosis. *Circled* area site best heard. *Shaded* area indicates radiation.

   e. In very severe lesion, split second may be fixed
3. Pulmonic ejection sound
   a. High frequency sound after S_1
   b. Best heard with diaphragm chestpiece
   c. Heard on straight line from base left to epigastric area

 Listen now to pulmonic stenosis from a real heart. You are listening at base right with a diaphragm chestpiece firmly pressed.

EISENMENGER'S SYNDROME

Eisenmenger's syndrome is a name loosely applied to any condition with a **left-to-right shunt** such as ASD, VSD, and persistent ductus arteriosus that subsequently develops severe pulmonary vascular hypertension. The pulmonary vascular hypertension causes a left-to-right shunt to reverse and become a predominantly **right-to-left shunt**. Fortunately this condition is rarely seen today, since children undergo surgery before such changes occur. However, if surgical correction is not done and a right-to-left shunt does occur, the following auscultatory sounds would be heard.

The auscultatory findings of Eisenmenger's syndrome are:
1. T_1 loud closure (results from increased right ventricular pressure)
2. Pulmonic ejection sound
   a. High-frequency sound after S_1
   b. Best heard with diaphragm chestpiece
   c. Heard on straight line from base left to epigastric area
   d. P_2, which is loud and may also be palpable
3. Systolic ejection murmur
   a. Grade II to III/IV
   b. Mix of high and low frequencies
   c. Harsh quality
   d. Equally well heard with either bell or diaphragm
   e. Heard along LLSB (Figure 17-10)
4. Split second sound
   a. High frequency with loud P_2 component
   b. Best heard with diaphragm
   c. Best heard at base left
   d. Type of split second sound heard helps to differentiate between etiologies of Eisenmenger's syndrome
      (1) Physiologically split second: consider persistent ductus arteriosus
      (2) Wide, fixed split second: consider ASD
      (3) Narrow, fixed split second: consider VSD

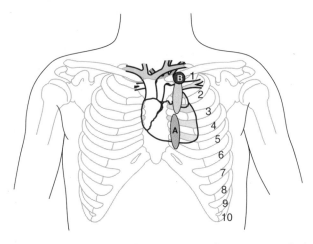

Figure 17-10   Eisenmenger's syndrome. **A,** Systolic murmur radiation; **B,** *circled* area site diastolic murmur best heard. *Shaded* area indicates radiation of diastolic murmur.

5. Diastolic murmur (pulmonary regurgitation resulting from failure of the pulmonary cusps to seal on closure)
   a. Lower frequency
   b. Rough in quality
   c. Best heard with bell chestpiece lightly held
   d. Best heard at base left and along upper LLSB (see Figure 17-10)

 Listen now to Eisenmenger's syndrome from a real heart. You are listening at base left with a diaphragm chestpiece firmly pressed.

TETRALOGY OF FALLOT (TOF)

Tetralogy of Fallot is the most common congenital lesion that produces cyanosis. In this pathologic condition there are various degrees of (1) pulmonary valvular stenosis, or infundibular stenosis, that result in decreased pulmonary blood flow; (2) a ventricular septal defect (VSD) with a right-to-left shunt; (3) an aorta that overrides the VSD; and (4) right ventricular hypertrophy. When the pulmonic stenosis is very severe, most of the blood is ejected through the ventricular septal defect. (See discussion on VSD in the following section for more information on the auscultatory sounds of this pathologic condition.) A common surgical procedure to correct a tetralogy of Fallot is the Blalock-Taussig operation. This correction causes a continuous murmur, which is explained in Chapter 19.

The pulmonary valvular stenosis or infundibular stenosis is the most common pathologic condition. The auscultatory findings for tetralogy of Fallot include:

1. Systolic murmur (ejection or pansystolic in nature, depending on the degree of pulmonic stenosis)
   a. Mix of high and low frequencies
   b. Rough quality
   c. Equally well heard with either bell or diaphragm
   d. Loudest in third or fourth left ICS (Figure 17-11)
   e. There is an inverse relationship between loudness of murmur and severity of condition
      (1) Murmur louder with moderate stenosis
      (2) Murmur soft to absent with very severe stenosis
2. P_2 component of the second sound
   a. Very soft and therefore, second sound perceived as single
   b. Physiological split second sound not heard
3. Aortic ejection sound may be present
   a. High frequency sound after S_1
   b. Best heard with diaphragm firmly pressed
   c. Heard on straight line from base right to apex

 Listen now to tetralogy of Fallot from a real heart. You are listening at the third to fourth left ICS with a diaphragm chestpiece firmly pressed.

VENTRICULAR SEPTAL DEFECT (SMALL)

The **ventricular septal defect** (VSD) that results from a hole in the ventricular septum is the most common pathologic condition associated

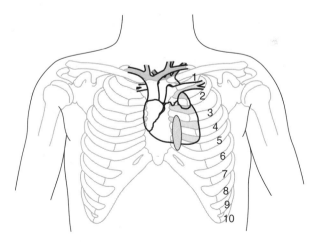

Figure 17-11   Tetralogy of Fallot. *Shaded* area indicates where heard.

with a systolic murmur in children. The direction of blood flow through the defect depends on the degree of pulmonary vascular outflow obstruction from either pulmonary stenosis or pulmonary hypertension. When this pulmonary outflow resistance is low, the flow is left to right; when this resistance is high, the flow is right to left. The murmur of the VSD depends on its size, position, and loudness.

The auscultatory findings of a small defect or one that is in the muscular septum are: (No diastolic murmur is heard.)

1. Systolic ejection murmur
   a. Small defect
      (1) High frequency
      (2) Mild harshness quality
      (3) Best heard with diaphragm firmly pressed
   b. Loud murmur
      (1) High frequency
      (2) Harsher quality
      (3) Best heard with either bell or diaphragm
   c. Best heard in third or fourth ICS to left of sternum (Figure 17-12)
   d. Radiation depends on the murmur's intensity
      (1) Very loud murmurs may be heard over entire precordium and on back
      (2) Usually are not heard in neck
2. Physiological split second may be heard
   a. High frequency
   b. Best heard with diaphragm firmly pressed
   c. Best heard at base left
3. Ejection sound absent

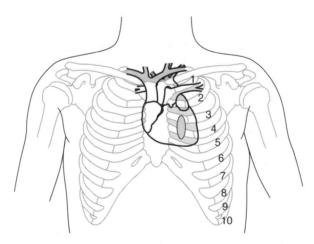

Figure 17-12   Ventricular septal defect (small). *Shaded* area indicates where heard.

4. The degree of pulmonary hypertension present has a significant influence on the auscultatory findings in VSD
   a. With slight pulmonary hypertension
      (1) Left-to-right shunt becomes smaller
      (2) Murmur becomes softer
   b. With more severe pulmonary hypertension
      (1) Left-to-right shunt is decreased
      (2) Systolic murmur may disappear
   c. With very severe pulmonary hypertension
      (1) Shunt changes right to left
      (2) Cyanosis is manifested
      (3) Eisenmenger's syndrome is manifested (See discussion of this syndrome, p. 139, for auscultatory findings.)

 Listen now to a VSD from a real heart. You are listening at the third to fourth left ICS with a diaphragm chestpiece firmly pressed.

SELF-LEARNING "UNKNOWN" HEART SOUNDS

 On the audio program, listen to the "unknown" heart sounds and identify the sound. Compare your answers with the answer key at the end of the chapter. Relisten to the audio program as needed to achieve mastery of the content.

You are listening to a real heart over the right ventricle between LLSB and the apex. You hear a systolic murmur that has a groaning, twanging quality and is heard equally well with either the bell or diaphragm chestpiece.

1. You identify the murmur as:
   a. arterial supraclavicular bruit
   b. physiologic systolic ejection murmur
   c. Still's murmur
   d. ASD

You are listening to a real heart of a 10-year-old at base right. The harsh murmur radiates to the apex and bilaterally into the neck. You hear the sound equally well with either a bell or diaphragm chestpiece.

2. You identify the murmur as:
   a. mitral valve prolapse   **b.** mitral regurgitation
   c. pulmonic stenosis   **d.** aortic stenosis

SELF-LEARNING QUESTIONS

1. List two of the physical findings common to those with an innocent or benign murmur.
   a.
   b.

2. The most common innocent murmur is:
   a. arterial supraclavicular bruit
   b. innocent pulmonary flow murmur
   c. Still's murmur
   d. mammary soufflé

3. The most common pathologic condition that causes a systolic murmur in a child is:
   a. Still's murmur
   b. physiologic systolic ejection murmur
   c. atrial septal defect
   d. ventricular septal defect

ANSWERS TO SELF-LEARNING "UNKNOWN" HEART SOUNDS

1. c

2. d

ANSWERS TO SELF-LEARNING QUESTIONS

1. Any two of the following: precordial activity is normal; first heart sound is normal; second heart sound splits physiologically; systolic murmur decreases in intensity on standing

2. c

3. d

C·H·A·P·T·E·R

18

Pediatric Diastolic Murmurs

LEARNING OBJECTIVES

After reading this chapter, listening to the accompanying audio program, answering the self-learning questions at the end of the chapter, and listening to the "unknowns" on the audio program, the learner will be able to do the following in infants and children:

1. Differentiate diastolic from systolic murmur.
2. Distinguish aortic valve regurgitation from pulmonic valve regurgitation.
3. Distinguish mitral valve stenosis from tricuspid valve stenosis.

DIASTOLIC MURMURS

Diastolic murmurs in children are not considered normal and always warrant an evaluation by a cardiologist. The origin of the diastolic murmur may be mitral or tricuspid valve stenosis (rare in children), aortic or pulmonic regurgitation, or as a part of a continuous murmur such as patent ductus arteriosus (PDA). Pathologic conditions having **only a diastolic murmur** are discussed in this chapter. Those as a part of a continuous murmur are discussed in Chapter 19.

AORTIC VALVE REGURGITATION

The most common etiology of **aortic valve regurgitation** in a child is a bicuspid aortic valve. Other causes include other congenital defects of the valve, acute rheumatic fever, or association with a high ventricular septal defect (VSD). When congenital, the murmur may be so soft at birth that it is missed or mistaken for breath sounds. As the child grows, the murmur may increase and become more discernible.

The auscultatory findings of aortic valve regurgitation include:
1. Softer than normal S_1
2. Aortic ejection sound (heard in congenital defect and not rheumatic cause)
   a. High frequency sound after S_1
   b. Best heard with diaphragm
   c. Heard on straight line from base right to apex
3. Early diastolic murmur
   a. Blowing quality
   b. Best heard with diaphragm firmly pressed
   c. Best heard at Erb's point
   d. Radiates down left sternal border or to apex. May radiate to back between fourth and eighth vertebral bodies to left of midline (Figure 18-1)
   e. Having patient sit up and lean forward in deep exhalation or lean back on elbows brings out this soft murmur

 Listen now to aortic valve regurgitation from a real heart. You are listening over Erb's point with a diaphragm chestpiece firmly pressed. The child is leaning forward.

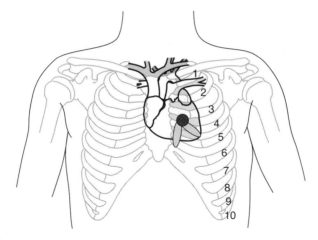

Figure 18-1   Aortic valve regurgitation. *Circled* area site best heard. *Shaded* area indicates radiation.

PULMONIC VALVE REGURGITATION

In children the surgical repair for tetralogy of Fallot may result in a **pulmonic valve regurgitation**, or it may result from a congenital defect of the pulmonic valve, pulmonary hypertension, or any infectious endocarditis.

The auscultatory findings of pulmonic valve regurgitation include:
1. Softer than normal S_1
2. Pulmonic ejection sound (heard in congenital defect and not rheumatic cause)
   a. High frequency sound after S_1
   b. Best heard with diaphragm
   c. Heard on straight line from base left and down to epigastrium
3. Early diastolic murmur
   a. Murmur of pulmonary hypertension
      (1) Starts just after S_2 and has long decrescendo extending to S_1
      (2) Medium pitched
      (3) Heard equally well with bell or diaphragm
   b. Best heard at base left and down upper left sternal border. May radiate to back between fourth and fifth thoracic vertebrae to left and right of spine (Figure 18-2)
   c. Murmur without pulmonary hypertension

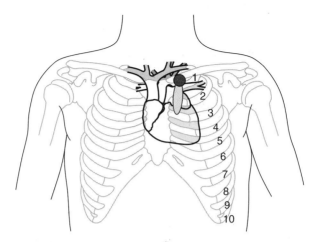

Figure 18-2   Pulmonic valve regurgitation. *Circled* area site best heard. *Shaded* area indicates radiation.

     (1) Starts slightly after S_2 and has short decrescendo
     (2) Lower pitched
     (3) Best heard with bell lightly held

 Listen now to the sounds of pulmonic valve regurgitation as recorded from a real heart. You are listening at base left with a diaphragm firmly pressed.

MITRAL VALVE STENOSIS

Mitral valve stenosis may result from acute rheumatic fever, which may occur in children between the ages of 5 and 14 years. Children have the same classic auscultatory heart sounds as those of the adult.

    The auscultatory findings of mitral valve stenosis include:

1. Louder than normal first sound
   a. Mitral leaflets are wide open when closed by left ventricular contraction
   b. Audible closure of stenotic leaflets
2. Opening snap
   a. High frequency sound after S_2
   b. Best heard with diaphragm
   c. Heard at apex or left sternal border with diaphragm
   d. Uncommon in children
3. Middiastolic murmur
   a. Rumble quality

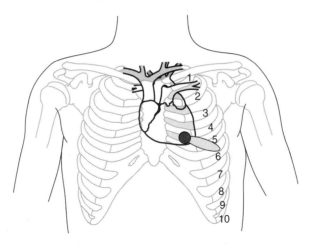

Figure 18-3   Mitral valve stenosis. *Circled* area site best heard. *Shaded* area indicates radiation.

      b. Best heard with bell lightly held
      c. Heard at apex with radiation to left axilla (Figure 18-3)
    4. Presystolic (late diastolic) accentuation of murmur
      a. Rumble quality
      b. Best heard with bell lightly held
      c. Heard at apex
      d. Radiates to left axilla

 Listen now to mitral valve stenosis from a real heart. You are listening at the apex with the bell chestpiece lightly held.

TRICUSPID VALVE STENOSIS

Tricuspid valve stenosis may also result from rheumatic fever and as such is generally associated with mitral valve stenosis.

    The auscultatory findings of tricuspid valve stenosis include:
    1. Louder than normal first sound
      a. Tricuspid leaflets are wide open when closed by left ventricular contraction
      b. Audible closure of stenotic leaflets
    2. Opening snap
      a. High frequency sound after S_2
      b. Best heard with diaphragm
      c. Best heard at lower end of sternum or lower right sternal border

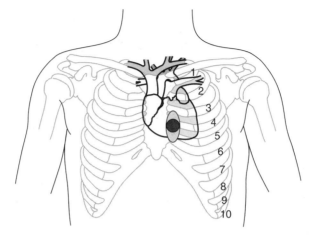

Figure 18-4   Tricuspid valve stenosis. *Circled* area site best heard. *Shaded* area indicates radiation.

    d. This audible opening of tricuspid valve stenosis is uncommon in children
3. Middiastolic murmur
    a. Rumble quality
    b. Best heard with bell lightly held
    c. Best heard at left sternal border with radiation along left sternal border (Figure 18-4)
4. Presystolic (late diastolic) accentuation of murmur
    a. Rumble quality
    b. Best heard with bell lightly held
    c. Best heard at left sternal border with radiation along left sternal border

 Listen now to tricuspid valve stenosis from a real heart. You are listening at left sternal border with the bell chestpiece lightly held.

SELF-LEARNING "UNKNOWN" HEART SOUNDS

 On the audio program, listen to the "unknown" heart sounds and identify the sound. Compare your answers with the answer key at the end of the chapter. Relisten to the audio program as needed to achieve mastery of the content.

You are listening at the apex with a bell lightly held.

1. You identify the pathologic condition as:
   a. mitral valve stenosis
   b. tricuspid valve stenosis
   c. aortic valve regurgitation
   d. pulmonic valve regurgitation

You are listening at Erb's point with a diaphragm firmly pressed. The child is leaning forward.

2. You identify the pathologic condition as:
   a. mitral valve stenosis
   b. tricuspid valve stenosis
   c. aortic valve regurgitation
   d. pulmonic valve regurgitation

SELF-LEARNING QUESTIONS

1. Diastolic murmurs in a child younger than 2 years may be considered normal.
   a. true
   b. false

2. The most common etiology of aortic valve regurgitation in a child is:
   a. rheumatic fever
   b. ventricular septal defect
   c. bicuspid aortic valve
   d. none of the above

3. The most common age for rheumatic fever in a child, which may result in mitral valve stenosis is:
   a. 1-2 months
   b. 6-9 months
   c. 1-3 years
   d. 5-14 years

ANSWERS TO SELF-LEARNING "UNKNOWN" HEART SOUNDS

1. a

2. c

ANSWERS TO SELF-LEARNING QUESTIONS

1. a

2. c

3. d

19

Pediatric Murmurs With Both Systolic and Diastolic Components

LEARNING OBJECTIVES

After reading this chapter, listening to the accompanying audio program, answering the self-learning questions at the end of the chapter, and listening to the "unknowns" on the audio program, the learner will be able to do the following in infants and children:

1. Identify an innocent murmur with a continuous sound.
2. Identify a pathologic condition that results when the functional closure of the ductus arteriosus fails to occur at birth.
3. Identify auscultatory findings heard after the Blalock-Taussig correction of tetralogy of Fallot.

CONTINUOUS MURMURS

Sustained noises that begin in systole and continue through the second heart sound into all or part of diastole are known as **continuous murmurs**. Most continuous murmurs with the exception of mammary soufflé and the cervical venous hum are pathological. Continuous murmurs can occur because of rapid blood flow, high-to-low pressure shunting, or localized arterial obstruction. The most common pediatric continuous murmurs are discussed in this chapter.

ATRIAL SEPTAL DEFECTS

An **atrial septal defect** (ASD) is a congenital cardiac anomaly characterized by an abnormal opening between the two atria. Of all congenital heart diseases seen in infancy, 10% to 15% are ASDs. Females are more commonly affected than are males. The three types of ASDs are (1) ostium primum, (2) ostium secundum, and (3) sinus venosus. The auscultatory findings in ASD vary, depending on the specific defect.

Ostium Primum ASD

Ostium primum ASD is a congenital opening low in the atrial septum, straddling the atrial-ventricular valves. Frequently a cleft is present in the aortic leaflet of the mitral valve in this defect. It is also known as an *endocardial cushion defect.*

The auscultatory features of ostium primum ASD include:
1. Systolic ejection murmur
   a. Grade II/VI
   b. Rumble quality
   c. Best heard with bell lightly held
   d. Heard at upper (second to third intercostal space [ICS]) left sternal border (Figure 19-1)
   e. May radiate to back at fourth to fifth thoracic vertebrae to left and right of spine
2. Loud T_1 component of the first sound
   a. High frequency sound
   b. Best heard with diaphragm
   c. Heard at lower left lateral sternal border (LLSB)
3. P_2 component of second sound
   a. Delayed because of increased volumes in right ventricle
   b. Loud with wide fixed splitting of S_2
   c. High frequency
   d. Best heard with diaphragm

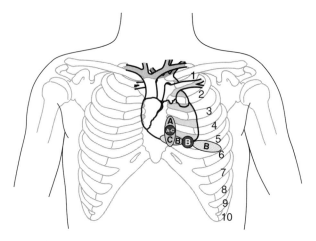

Figure 19-1   Ostium primum atrial septal defect (ASD). *Circled* area site best heard. *Shaded* area indicates radiation. **A,** Site systolic rumble murmur best heard; **B,** site systolic blow of mitral regurgitation best heard; **C,** site diastolic rumble murmur best heard.

      e. Heard at base left
   4. Systolic murmur if mitral valve regurgitation occurs through cleft in anterior cusp of mitral valve
      a. Late systolic with mild regurgitation
      b. Pansystolic with severe regurgitation
      c. Blowing quality
      d. Best heard with diaphragm firmly pressed
      e. Best heard at apex with radiation to left axilla and left sternal border; may radiate to back at fourth to fifth thoracic vertebrae to left and right of spine
   5. Short middiastolic murmur (with large shunt)
      a. Rumble quality
      b. Best heard with bell lightly held
      c. Heard along lower left sternal border (see Figure 19-1)
   6. When patient stands, all auscultatory features of ASD will still be present

Ostium Secundum ASD

Ostium secundum ASD is a congenital defect at the fossa ovalis caused by failure of development of septum secundum. Occasionally, especially in women, this ASD will persist into adulthood.

   The auscultatory features of ostium secundum ASD include:
   1. Systolic ejection murmur
      a. Grade II/VI

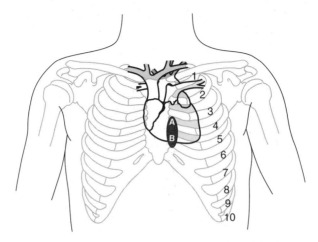

Figure 19-2   Sinus venosus atrial septal defect (ASD) and ostium secundum ASD. **A,** Site systolic murmur best heard; **B,** site diastolic murmur best heard.

      b. Rumble quality
      c. Best heard with bell lightly held
      d. Heard at upper (second to third ICS) left sternal border (Figure 19-2)
  2. Short middiastolic murmur
      a. Rumble quality
      b. Best heard with bell lightly held
      c. Heard along lower left sternal border (see Figure 19-2)
  3. T_1 component of first sound is loud
      a. High frequency
      b. Best heard with diaphragm
      c. Best heard at LLSB
  4. P_2 is delayed and loud with wide fixed splitting of S_2
      a. High frequency
      b. Heard with diaphragm firmly pressed
      c. Heard at base left
  5. When patient stands, all auscultatory features of ASD will still be present

Sinus Venosus ASD

Sinus venosus ASD is a defect posterior to fossa ovalis and one that occurs high in the atrial septum because of maldevelopment of part of the sinus venosus. It is always associated with anomalous pulmonary venous connection of the right superior pulmonary vein to the lower end of the superior vena cava with drainage of the right lung into the right atrium.

The auscultatory features of sinus venosus ASD include:

1. Systolic ejection murmur
   a. Grade II/VI
   b. Rumble quality
   c. Best heard with bell chestpiece lightly held
   d. Heard at upper (second to third ICS) left sternal border (see Figure 19-2)
2. Diastolic flow murmur (caused by increased flow through normal tricuspid valve)
   a. Grade II/VI
   b. Rumble quality
   c. Best heard with bell chestpiece lightly held
   d. Heard along lower left sternal border (see Figure 19-2)
3. Wide split S_2
   a. Wide during expiration
   b. Widens further on inspiration
   c. High frequency
   d. Best heard with diaphragm firmly pressed
   e. Heard at base left
4. When patient stands, all auscultatory features of ASD will still be present

 Listen now to an ostium secundum ASD from a real heart. You are listening along the lower left sternal border with a bell chestpiece lightly held.

CERVICAL VENOUS HUM

The **cervical venous hum** is the second most common **innocent** murmur of toddlers to school-age children. The "hum" is produced by turbulence in the blood flow in the internal jugular vein as blood flows from the head and neck into the thorax.

The auscultatory findings of cervical venous hum are:

1. Continuous sound with accentuation during diastole
   a. Low in frequency and soft
   b. Best heard with bell chestpiece lightly held
   c. Heard continuously just above clavicle on both right and left sides but more commonly heard on right when child is sitting (Figure 19-3)
   d. May radiate slightly down sternum, but this radiation is rare
   e. Loudest on sitting or standing
2. Hum obliterated by

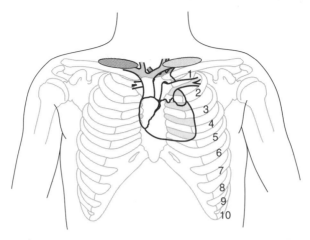

Figure 19-3   Cervical venous hum. *Shaded* area indicates where heard.

    a. Turning head
    b. Light pressure with finger over jugular vein
    c. Lying supine
    d. Valsalva maneuver also usually stops hum
  3. Hum increased in conditions with increased blood flow
    a. Thyrotoxicosis
    b. Anemia
  4. Does not require referral to pediatric cardiologist
  5. Differential diagnoses include
    a. Patent ductus arteriosus (PDA)
    b. Atrial-ventricular (A-V) fistula
    c. This differentiation is easy because
      (1) Hum can be silenced by the maneuvers just described
      (2) PDA and A-V fistula remain audible with these maneuvers

 Listen now to a cervical venous hum from a real heart. You are listening just above the right clavicle with a bell chestpiece lightly held.

MAMMARY SOUFFLÉ

The **mammary soufflé** is an **innocent** murmur that may be heard in the latter months of pregnancy or during lactation. It seems to be caused by increased blood flow in the internal mammary and intercostal arteries. Because girls younger than 18 years may become pregnant, this murmur is included under innocent murmurs of childhood.

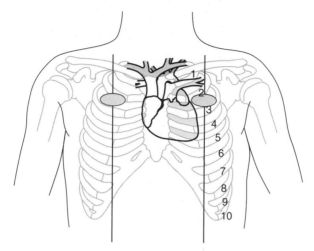

Figure 19-4   Mammary soufflé. *Shaded* area indicates where heard.

The auscultatory findings of mammary soufflé include:
1. Systolic ejection murmur
    a. High pitched
    b. Best heard with diaphragm chestpiece
    c. Best heard over or just above breasts in second right or left ICS in midclavicular line and has very little radiation (Figure 19-4)
    d. Most obvious when lying flat and decreases with upright posture or pressure with stethoscope over area
2. May have diastolic component
    a. High pitched
    b. Best heard with diaphragm chestpiece
    c. Best heard over or just above breasts in second right or left ICS in midclavicular line and has very little radiation
    d. Most obvious when lying flat and decreases with upright posture or pressure with stethoscope over area
3. Does not require referral to pediatric cardiologist
4. Obliteration of this murmur with pressure permits differentiation of this murmur from that of patent ductus arteriosus

PATENT DUCTUS ARTERIOSUS

A **patent ductus arteriosus** (PDA) results when the functional closure of the ductus arteriosus fails to occur at birth. In fetal life the ductus arteriosus connects the pulmonary artery to the aorta and shunts oxygenated blood directly into the systemic circulation, bypassing the lungs. Normal closure occurs a few hours after birth, although complete

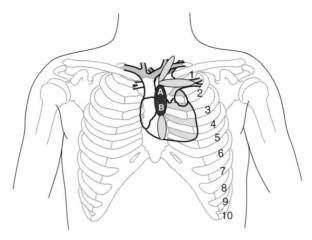

Figure 19-5   Patent ductus arteriosus (PDA). **A,** *Circled* area site systolic murmur best heard; **B,** *circled* area site diastolic murmur best heard. *Shaded* area indicates radiation of murmurs.

closure may take several weeks. The cardiac findings of a PDA depend on the size of the ductus and the pulmonary vascular resistance and depend on the dynamic relationship between the pulmonary and systemic vascular beds, which can change from moment to moment.

An auscultatory hallmark of PDA is a continuous "to and fro" or "machinery-like" murmur with both a systolic and diastolic component. Because pressure in the aorta is higher than in the pulmonary arteries both in systole and diastole, turbulent blood flow continues whether aortic or pulmonic valve is open or closed. The blood flowing from the aorta through the patent ductus to the pulmonary artery causes the murmur. Infants with significant PDA usually have a wide pulse pressure with bounding peripheral pulses.

The auscultatory findings in PDA are:
1. Continuous "to and fro" or "machinery-like" murmur
   a. Both systolic and diastolic component
   b. Harsh quality
   c. Equally well heard with either bell or diaphragm chestpiece
   d. Best heard at middle to upper left sternal border (Figure 19-5)
   e. Radiates widely to left infraclavicular area, neck, and along left sternal border
   f. Initially murmur may be absent in neonates or premature infants, who have a normally high pulmonary resistance that tends to equalize the pressure between the two vessels
   g. After exercise, the continuous murmur becomes more pronounced

2. S$_3$ (pathological S$_3$ if congestive heart failure [CHF] is component of PDA)
   a. Low frequency
   b. Best heard with bell chestpiece lightly held
   c. Best heard at apex
3. S$_4$ (may also be heard if CHF is component of PDA)
   a. Low frequency
   b. Best heard with bell chestpiece lightly held
   c. Best heard at apex

The auscultatory findings of a small PDA may include:
1. Systolic ejection murmur only with no diastolic murmur
   a. Blowing quality
   b. Best heard with diaphragm chestpiece firmly pressed
   c. Best heard at middle to upper left sternal border
   d. Murmurs of small VSD do not radiate to back
2. Differential diagnoses include
   a. VSD
   b. Peripheral pulmonary stenosis
   c. High output states

 Listen now to a patent ductus arteriosus from a real heart. You are listening at the middle to upper left sternal border with either a bell or diaphragm chestpiece.

VENTRICULAR SEPTAL DEFECT (LARGE)

Ventricular septal defect (VSD) is a defect in the interventricular septal wall, most often in the membranous (upper portion) ventricular septum. Small defects may close spontaneously. Because there is little flow through the defect until the pulmonary vascular resistance found at birth falls, the defect may not be detected until 6 weeks of age when sufficient blood flows through the defect to cause a murmur. The auscultatory findings of the VSD, especially the murmur, depend on its size, position, and loudness.

The auscultatory findings in a small VSD with diastolic murmur are:
1. Pansystolic murmur
   a. Soft intensity
      (1) Higher frequency
      (2) Mild harshness quality
      (3) Best heard with diaphragm firmly pressed
      (4) Best heard in third to fourth intercostal space (ICS) to left of sternum (Figure 19-6)
      (5) Radiation to entire precordium

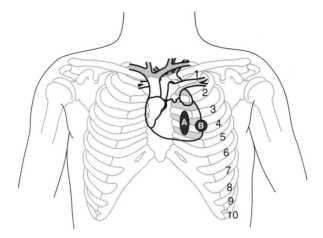

Figure 19-6   Ventricular septal defect (large). **A,** Site systolic murmur best heard; **B,** site diastolic murmur best heard.

   b. Loud Intensity
      (1) Medium frequency
      (2) Harsher quality
      (3) Best heard with diaphragm firmly pressed
      (4) Best heard in third to fourth ICS to left of sternum
      (5) Radiates to entire precordium and on the back; they usually are not heard in the neck
2. Physiological split second or widely split second
   a. High frequency
   b. Best heard with diaphragm firmly pressed
   c. Best heard at base left
3. Middiastolic flow murmur (may not be heard if shunt very small)
   a. Rumble quality
   b. Best heard with bell lightly held
   c. Best heard at apex (see Figure 19-6)
4. S$_3$ (when CHF present)
   a. Low frequency sound just after S$_2$
   b. Best heard with bell lightly held
   c. Best heard at apex
The auscultatory findings in a large VSD are:
1. Pansystolic murmur
   a. Harsh quality
   b. Heard equally well with bell or diaphragm
   c. Best heard in third to fourth ICS to left of sternum
   d. Radiation depends on murmur's intensity; very loud murmurs

may be heard over entire precordium and on back; they usually are not heard in neck

2. Physiological split second may be absent
3. Middiastolic flow murmur
   a. Rumble quality
   b. Best heard with bell lightly held
   c. Best heard at apex
4. S_3 (when CHF present)
   a. Low frequency sound just after S_2
   b. Best heard with bell lightly held
   c. Best heard at apex

The auscultatory sounds heard with marked pulmonary hypertension are:

1. Short systolic ejection murmur
   a. High frequency
   b. Best heard with diaphragm firmly pressed
   c. Heard at left sternal border
2. Wide split S_2 with loud P_2 component
   a. High frequency
   b. Best heard with diaphragm firmly pressed
   c. Heard at base left
3. When pulmonary vascular resistance exceeds systemic resistance, direction of shunt will be reversed and blood will flow from right to left ventricle (See Eisenmenger's syndrome in Chapter 17 for auscultatory findings.)

The auscultatory sounds heard when the defect is in the muscular septum are (during systole, muscular contraction may close defect or the tricuspid valve may occlude it):

1. Early systolic murmur
   a. High frequency
   b. Best heard with diaphragm firmly pressed
   c. Heard at left sternal border
2. Diastolic murmur not heard

 Listen now to a large VSD from a real heart. You are listening at third to fourth ICS to the left of the sternum with either a bell or diaphragm chestpiece.

BLALOCK-TAUSSIG CORRECTION OF TETRALOGY OF FALLOT

This procedure is a surgical construction of a shunt as a temporary measure to overcome congenital pulmonary valve stenosis and atrial septal defect. It creates an end-to-side subclavian artery to pulmonary artery shunt.

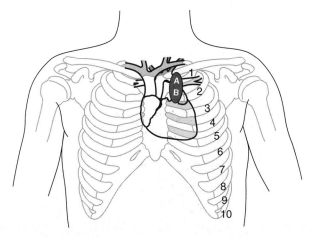

Figure 19-7   Blalock-Taussig correction of tetralogy of Fallot (TOF). **A,** Site systolic murmur best heard; **B,** site diastolic murmur best heard.

The auscultatory sounds present after this procedure are:
1. Continuous murmur heard in systole and diastole
   a. High in frequency
   b. Blowing quality
   c. Best heard with diaphragm firmly pressed
   d. Heard under clavicle on side of shunt and over operative scar (Figure 19-7)
2. If shunt is small or pulmonary vascular resistance high as in large shunt
   a. Systolic murmur only
   b. Diastolic murmur not heard
3. If shunt narrows or is occluding
   a. Murmur changes over time
   b. Systolic component only
   c. Diastolic component is lost

 Listen now to the continuous murmur of the Blalock-Taussig shunt from a real heart. You are listening under the clavicle on the side of shunt and over the operative scar with a diaphragm chestpiece firmly pressed.

SELF-LEARNING "UNKNOWN" HEART SOUNDS

 On the audio program, listen to the "unknown" heart sounds and identify the sound. Compare your answers with the answer key at the end of the chapter. Relisten to the audio program as needed to achieve mastery of the content.

You are listening to a real heart above the right clavicle with a bell chestpiece lightly held.

1. You identify the sound as:
   a. cervical venous hum
   b. atrial septal defect (ostium secundum)
   c. patent ductus arteriosus (PDA)
   d. large VSD

You are listening to a real heart at the middle to upper left sternal border with either a bell or diaphragm chestpiece.

2. You identify the sound as:
   a. cervical venous hum
   b. atrial septal defect (ostium secundum)
   c. patent ductus arteriosus (PDA)
   d. large VSD

SELF-LEARNING QUESTIONS

1. The pathologic condition that results when the functional closure of the ductus arteriosus fails to occur at birth is:
   a. VSD   b. ASD
   c. PDA   d. none of the above

2. The murmur that is best heard under the clavicle on the side of a shunt and over the operative scar with a diaphragm chestpiece firmly pressed is that of:
   a. ostium primum ASD
   b. patent ductus arteriosus
   c. cervical venous hum
   d. Blalock-Taussig correction of TOF

3. The ostium primum is a type of:
   a. VSD   b. ASD
   c. PDA   d. none of the above

ANSWERS TO SELF-LEARNING "UNKNOWN" HEART SOUNDS

1. a

2. b

ANSWERS TO SELF-LEARNING QUESTIONS

1. c

2. d

3. b

20

When To Refer

LEARNING OBJECTIVES

After reading this chapter and answering the self-learning questions at the end of the chapter, the learner will be able to do the following in infants and children:

1. Identify percentage of school-age children with an innocent murmur.
2. Identify two reasons not to refer a child with a murmur to a pediatric cardiologist.
3. Identify two reasons to refer a child with a murmur to a pediatric cardiologist.

OVERALL MURMUR PREVALENCE

It is estimated that 2% to 57% of infants and 6% to 90% of school-age children will have innocent murmurs. Innocent murmurs are ten times more common than pathological ones.
1. Innocent murmurs
   a. Still's murmur most common
   b. Venous hum second most common
2. Pathological murmurs
   a. Ventricular septal defect (VSD): 38%
   b. Atrial septal defect (ASD): 18%
   c. Pulmonary valve stenosis: 13%
   d. Pulmonary artery stenosis: 7%
   e. Aortic valve stenosis: 4%
   f. Patent ductus arteriosus (PDA): 4%
   g. Mitral valve prolapse: 4%
   h. Others: 12%

DIFFERENTIATING INNOCENT MURMURS FROM PATHOLOGICAL MURMURS

Innocent murmurs should always accompany a normal history, physical examination, and appearance without symptoms. Although two of the innocent murmurs may be of continuous types, cervical venous hum and mammary soufflé, they are never solely diastolic. When attempting to determine whether a murmur is innocent or pathological, the examiner should consider the following signs of an innocent murmur:
1. Normal precordial activity
2. Timing is systolic or continuous
3. Area of maximal intensity is well localized
4. Grade is either I/VI or II/VI; always less than III/VI
5. Second sound splits physiologically
6. Innocent systolic murmur decreases with standing
7. Innocent murmur may intensify with fever, activity, anemia, or stress
8. Other physiological features contributing to innocent murmurs
   a. Thin chest wall in children
   b. More angulated great vessels in children
   c. More dynamic circulation in children

Pathological murmurs may be found in a symptomatic child with an abnormal history, physical examination, or appearance. The presence of cyanosis should always make one suspicious of congenital heart disease. Signs of pathological murmurs include:

1. Abnormal precordial activity
2. Evidence of failure to thrive
3. Lethargy
4. Cyanosis
5. Shortness of breath
6. Auscultatory signs
   a. Harsh murmur
   b. Diastolic murmur only
   c. Pansystolic murmur
   d. Grade III/VI or greater
   e. Area of maximal intensity is diffuse
   f. Murmur radiates to back or neck
   g. Abnormal split of second sound
   h. Pathological murmur increases with standing

WHEN TO REFER

Because most children have an audible murmur at some point from infancy to adolescence, it is important for a practitioner to be able to differentiate innocent from pathological murmurs. Unnecessary referrals to a pediatric cardiologist are not only anxiety producing for the family but also costly. Auscultation of the heart is the most effective method for assessing murmurs.

A cardiac pathologic condition should be suspected when infants have poor feeding, failure to thrive, or unexplained respiratory symptoms or cyanosis. These may be signs of congenital heart disease. All patients should be carefully evaluated for these signs or symptoms. Patients with a suspected cardiac pathologic condition should be referred to a pediatric cardiologist for evaluation. Patients with an innocent murmur will not have such signs and will be asymptomatic. The patient who manifests signs of an innocent murmur may be followed by a primary care practitioner.

Unstable or acutely ill children with a suspected cardiac pathologic condition should be referred urgently. In older children, indicators of possible serious cardiac disease include chest pain, especially with exercise; dizziness; or syncope. Congestive heart failure (CHF) is another indicator of cardiac disease. Infants may manifest CHF with tachypnea, tachycardia, cardiomegalia, wheezing, weak peripheral pulses, poor feeding, poor weight gain, and diaphoresis. Children have similar signs with the addition of dyspnea on exertion, peripheral edema, and decreased urine output.

The murmur of atrial septal defect (ASD) may be easily mistaken for an innocent murmur.

SELF-LEARNING QUESTIONS

1. The percentage of school-age children who can have an innocent murmur is as high as:
   a. 5%   b. 15%
   c. 50%   d. 90%

2. List two reasons why you would not refer a child with a murmur to a pediatric cardiologist.
   a.
   b.

3. List two reasons why you would refer a child with a murmur to a pediatric cardiologist.
   a.
   b.

ANSWERS TO SELF-LEARNING QUESTIONS

1. d

2. No referral is necessary for any of the following:
   a. Innocent murmur with normal history and without symptoms
   b. Normal precordial activity
   c. Timing is systolic or continuous
   d. Area of maximal intensity is well localized
   e. Grade is usually I/VI or II/VI; always less than III/VI
   f. Second sound splits physiologically
   g. Innocent systolic murmur decreases with standing
   h. Innocent murmur may intensify with fever, activity, anemia, or stress
   i. Other physiological features contributing to innocent murmurs
      (1) Thin chest wall in children
      (2) More angulated great vessels in children
      (3) More dynamic circulation in children

2. Referral is necessary for any of the following:
   a. Symptomatic children with abnormal history
   b. Abnormal precordial activity
   c. Evidence of failure to thrive
   d. Lethargy
   e. Cyanosis

   f. Shortness of breath

   g. Auscultatory signs

      (1) Harsh murmur

      (2) Diastolic murmur only

      (3) Pansystolic murmur

      (4) Grade III/VI or greater

      (5) Area of maximal intensity is diffuse

      (6) Murmur radiates to back or neck

      (7) Abnormal split of second sound

      (8) Pathological murmur increases with standing

Appendix
Transcript for Audio Program

CHAPTER 2: THE FIRST HEART SOUND

Listen now to a sound that is split at various distances. A split of .08 seconds . . . split of .06 seconds . . . split of .04 seconds . . . split of .02 seconds . . . single sound . . . split .02 seconds . . . single sound . . . split .02 seconds . . .

Listen now to a normal heart sound at the various sites. First sound: left lateral sternal border, split . . . first sound: left lateral sternal border, single . . . apex, single first sound . . . base right, single first sound . . . base left, single first sound . . . Intensity of the first sound. Loud sound followed by soft sound . . . soft sound followed by loud sound . . .

Listen to the normal first sound at various sites. Left lateral sternal border, first sound slightly louder than the second sound . . . apex, first sound slightly louder than the second sound . . . base right, first sound slightly softer than the second sound . . .

When listening to a normal first sound, the following is normal for the sites specified: left lateral sternal border, first sound single slightly louder than the second sound . . . left lateral sternal border, first sound split slightly louder than the second sound . . . apex, first sound single louder than the second . . . base right, first sound single softer than the second . . . base left, first sound single softer than the second . . .

Self-Learning "Unknown" Heart Sounds—Chapter 2

"Unknown" No. 1 . . .
"Unknown" No. 2 . . .
"Unknown" No. 3 . . .
"Unknown" No. 4 . . .
"Unknown" No. 5 . . .

CHAPTER 3: THE SECOND HEART SOUND (S_2)

Listen now to a physiological split second sound. The split is audible on inspiration, the sound single on expiration . . . expiration . . . inspiration . . . expiration . . . inspiration . . . expiration . . . Listen again to a second sound that is split and a second sound that is single. A second sound split . . . a second sound single . . .

Listen now to a normal second sound at the various auscultatory sites: left lateral sternal border, single second sound . . . apex, single second sound . . . base right, single second sound . . . base left, physiological split second sound . . . inspiration . . . expiration . . . inspiration . . . expiration . . .

Listen to the loudness of the normal second sound at the various auscultatory sites: left lateral sternal border, second sound softer than the first . . . apex, second sound softer than the first . . . base right, second sound louder than the first . . . base left, second sound louder than the first . . .

When listening to the normal second sound, the following is normal for the sites specified: left lateral sternal border, second single sound softer than the first . . . apex, second sound single softer than the first . . . base right, second sound single louder than the first . . . base left, second sound splits on inspiration, single on expiration, louder than the first . . . inspiration . . . expiration . . . inspiration . . . expiration . . . inspiration . . . expiration . . .

Review now the normal first and second heart sounds for the sites specified: left lateral sternal border, single first, single second, first louder than the second . . . left lateral sternal border, split first, single second, first louder than the second . . . apex, single first, single second, first louder than the second . . . base right, single first, single second, first softer than the second . . . base left, single first, physiological split second, first softer than the second . . . inspiration . . . expiration . . . inspiration . . . expiration . . .

Self-Learning "Unknown" Heart Sounds—Chapter 3

"Unknown" No. 1 . . . inspiration . . . expiration . . . inspiration . . . expiration . . .
"Unknown" No. 2 . . . inspiration . . . expiration . . . inspiration . . . expiration . . .
"Unknown" No. 3 . . .
"Unknown" No. 4 . . .
"Unknown" No. 5 . . .

CHAPTER 4: THE FOURTH HEART SOUND (S_4)

Listen now to our fourth heart sound. Initially, only S_1 and S_2 will be heard, then an S_4 will be added . . . S_4 . . . S_4 out . . . S_4 . . .

Listen now to a heart with an S_4 with a bell lightly held. Then pressure will be put on the bell. Note that the S_4 disappears . . . bell lightly held . . . pressure on the bell . . . bell lightly held . . . pressure on the bell . . .

Differentiating S_4 from a split first sound . . . listen to an S_4 . . . bell lightly held . . . pressure on the bell . . . bell lightly held . . . pressure on the bell . . .

Listen now to a split S_1 . . . single first sound . . . split first sound . . . single first sound . . .

Again, listen to an S_4 compared to a split S_1 . . . S_4 . . . split first sound . . . single first sound . . . S_4 . . . single first sound . . . split first sound . . . split first sound with an S_4 in front of it . . . S_4 . . . single first sound . . . split first sound . . .

Self-Learning "Unknown" Heart Sounds—Chapter 4

"Unknown" No. 1: You are listening to the heart at the left lateral sternal border. Using the bell lightly held, you hear . . . using the bell firmly pressed, you hear . . . using the diaphragm, you hear . . .

"Unknown" No. 2: You are listening to the heart at the left lateral sternal border. Using the bell lightly held, you hear . . . using the bell firmly pressed, you hear . . . using the diaphragm, you hear . . .

"Unknown" No. 3: You are listening to the heart at the apex. Using the bell lightly held, you hear . . . using the bell firmly pressed, you hear . . . using the diaphragm, you hear . . .

"Unknown" No. 4: You are listening to the heart at the apex. Using the bell lightly held, you hear . . . using the bell firmly pressed, you hear . . . using the diaphragm, you hear . . .

"Unknown" No. 5: You are listening to the heart at the left lateral sternal border. Using the bell lightly held, you hear . . . using the bell firmly pressed, you hear . . . using the diaphragm, you hear . . .

CHAPTER 5: THE THIRD HEART SOUND (S_3)

Listen now to an S_3. Initially only S_1 and S_2 will be heard, then S_3 will be added . . . S_3 . . . S_1, S_2 . . . S_3 . . .

Differentiating S_3 from S_4. Timing permits the S_3 to be distinguished from the S_4. S_3 comes after the S_2 . . . S_4 comes before the S_1 . . . single S_1 and S_2 . . . Listen again: S_3 after S_2 . . . S_4 before S_1 . . . single S_4 and S_2 . . . quadruple rhythm, S_4 in front of S_1, S_3 after S_2 . . . S_4 out . . . S_3 out . . . S_4 before S_1 . . . S_3 after S_2 . . . summation gallop, S_3 and S_4 at a rapid rate . . . S_3 and S_4 out . . . S_3 and S_4 in . . . S_3 and S_4 out . . . S_3 and S_4 in . . .

Self-Learning "Unknown" Heart Sounds—Chapter 5

"Unknown" No. 1: You are listening to the heart at the apex. Using the bell lightly held, you hear . . . using the bell firmly pressed, you hear . . . using the diaphragm, you hear . . .

"Unknown" No. 2: You are listening to the heart at base left during inspiration.

Using the bell lightly held, you hear . . . using the bell firmly pressed, you hear . . . using the diaphragm, you hear . . .

"Unknown" No. 3: You are listening to the heart at the apex. Using the bell lightly held, you hear . . . using the bell firmly pressed, you hear . . . using the diaphragm, you hear . . .

"Unknown" No. 4: You are listening to the heart at the apex. Using the bell lightly held, you hear . . . using the bell firmly pressed, you hear . . . using the diaphragm, you hear . . .

"Unknown" No. 5: You are listening to the heart at the apex. Using the bell lightly held, you hear . . . using the bell firmly pressed, you hear . . . using the diaphragm, you hear . . .

CHAPTER 6: MURMURS—GENERAL INFORMATION

Listen now to murmurs that are considered high, medium, and low in frequency, heard equally well with either bell or diaphragm . . . low frequency, heard best with the bell lightly held . . .

Listen now to murmurs that are described as "blowing," "harsh" or "rough," and "rumble." First, listen to a blowing murmur, mainly high frequency . . . now a harsh or rough murmur, mainly medium frequencies . . . now a rumble, mainly low frequencies . . .

Listen now to a heart beating 60 times per minute. First, a systolic blow murmur will be added, then removed . . . systolic blow . . . systolic blow gone . . . systolic blow . . . systolic blow gone . . .

Listen now to a diastolic rumble. It will be added and removed . . . diastolic rumble . . . diastolic rumble gone . . . diastolic rumble . . . diastolic rumble gone . . .

Listen now to a heart beating 60 times per minute. Then a murmur will be added in the systolic period, early, mid, late, and pan. Early systolic murmur . . . midsystolic murmur . . . late systolic murmur . . . pansystolic murmur . . .

Listen now to a heart beating 60 times per minute. Then a murmur will be added in the diastolic period, early, mid, late, and pandiastolic. First, an early diastolic . . . middiastolic murmur . . . late diastolic murmur . . . pandiastolic murmur . . .

Self-Learning "Unknown" Heart Sounds—Chapter 6

Determine the frequency of the following sustained sounds:

"Unknown" No. 1: This sound is heard best with the diaphragm firmly pressed . . .

"Unknown" No. 2: This sound is heard equally well with either the bell or the diaphragm . . .

"Unknown" No. 3: This sound is heard best with the bell lightly held . . .

"Unknown" No. 4: This sound is heard best with the diaphragm firmly pressed . . .
"Unknown" No. 5: This sound is heard best with the bell lightly held . . .

CHAPTER 7: SYSTOLIC MURMURS

Listen now to a heart beating 60 times per minute. Then an early systolic murmur will be added . . .

Listen now to a heart beating 60 times per minute. Then an early innocent murmur will be added. The early murmur will then be compared to the one that is midsystolic in type . . . early . . . mid . . .

Listen now to a heart beating 60 times per minute. Then a midsystolic murmur will be added, which is medium in frequency and harsh in quality . . .

Listen now to a heart beating 60 times per minute. Then a late systolic murmur will be added, which is high in frequency, blowing in quality . . .

Listen now to a heart beating 60 times per minute. Then a pansystolic or holosystolic murmur will be added, which is high in frequency and blowing in quality . . .

Self-Learning "Unknown" Heart Sounds—Chapter 7

"Unknown" No. 1 . . .
"Unknown" No. 2 . . .
"Unknown" No. 3 . . .
"Unknown" No. 4 . . .
"Unknown" No. 5 . . .

CHAPTER 8: DIASTOLIC MURMURS

Listen now to a heart beating 60 times per minute. Then an early diastolic murmur will be added, which is high in frequency and blowing in quality . . .

Listen now to a heart beating 60 times per minute. Then a middiastolic murmur will be added, which is low in frequency and rumbling in quality . . .

Listen now to a heart beating 60 times per minute. Then a late diastolic murmur will be added, which is low in frequency and rumbling in quality . . .

Listen now to a heart beating 60 times per minute. Then a pandiastolic murmur is added, which is low in frequency and rumbling in quality . . .

Self-Learning "Unknown" Heart Sounds—Chapter 8

Listen to the following diastolic murmurs:
"Unknown" No. 1 . . .

"Unknown" No. 2 . . .
"Unknown" No. 3 . . .
"Unknown" No. 4 . . .
"Unknown" No. 5 . . .

CHAPTER 9: SOUNDS AROUND S₁

Listen to a wide split first sound as compared with a normal split first sound and a single first sound . . . single first sound . . . wide split first sound . . . single first sound . . . normal split first sound . . . single first sound . . . normal split first sound . . . wide split first sound . . . single first sound . . . normal split first sound . . . wide split first sound . . .

Pulmonic Ejection Sounds

Pulmonic ejection sound compared to the single first sound . . . single first sound . . . pulmonic ejection sound . . . single first sound . . . pulmonic ejection sound . . .

Aortic Ejection Sounds

Aortic ejection sound compared to single first sounds . . . single first sound . . . aortic ejection sounds . . . single first sound . . . aortic ejection sound . . .

Midsystolic Clicks

Midsystolic click compared to single first sound . . . single first sound . . . midsystolic click . . . single first sound . . . midsystolic click . . .

A midsystolic click will move closer to the first sound with standing . . . midsystolic click . . . standing . . . single first sound . . . midsystolic click . . . standing . . .

A midsystolic click will move farther from the first sound with squatting . . . midsystolic click . . . squatting . . . single first sound . . . midsystolic click . . . squatting . . .

Self-Learning "Unknown" Heart Sounds—Chapter 9

You are listening to the heart at base left, with the diaphragm firmly pressed. Unknown No. 1 . . .

"Unknown" No. 2: You are listening to a heart with the diaphragm firmly pressed at the left lateral sternal border, you hear . . . at the apex, you hear . . . at base right, you hear . . . at base left, you hear . . .

"Unknown" No. 3: You are listening to a heart with the diaphragm firmly pressed. At the left lateral sternal border, you hear . . . at the apex, you hear . . . at base right, you hear . . . at base left, you hear . . .

"Unknown" No. 4: You are listening to a heart with the diaphragm firmly pressed.

At the left lateral sternal border, you hear . . . at the apex, you hear . . . at base right, you hear . . . at base left, you hear . . .

"Unknown" No. 5: You are listening to the heart at the apex. Using the bell lightly held, you hear . . . using the bell firmly pressed, you hear . . . using the diaphragm, you hear . . .

CHAPTER 10: SOUNDS AROUND S$_2$

Listen now to a paradoxical second sound. The split is audible on expiration. The sound is single on inspiration . . . expiration . . . inspiration . . . expiration . . . inspiration . . .

Listen now to a wide split second compared to a single second sound . . . wide split second sound . . . normal split second sound . . . single second sound . . . wide split second sound . . . normal split second sound . . . single second sound . . .

Listen now to a fixed split second sound . . . fixed split second sound . . . inspiration . . . expiration . . . physiological split second sound . . . inspiration . . . expiration . . . inspiration . . . expiration . . .

Listen now to a narrow split second compared to a physiological split second . . . narrow split second sound . . . inspiration . . . expiration . . . inspiration . . . expiration . . . physiological split second sound . . . inspiration . . . expiration . . . inspiration . . . expiration . . .

Listen now to a second sound followed by an opening snap. The opening snap will be taken in and out . . . opening snap present . . . opening snap gone . . . opening snap present . . . opening snap gone . . .

Differentiating S$_3$ from the opening snap. First an opening snap will be heard . . . opening snap gone . . . S$_3$ . . . S$_3$ gone . . . opening snap . . . opening snap gone . . . S$_3$ . . . S$_3$ gone . . . opening snap . . . followed by S$_3$ . . .

Self-Learning "Unknown" Heart Sounds—Chapter 10

You are listening to the heart at base left, with the diaphragm firmly pressed.

"Unknown" No. 1 . . . inspiration . . . expiration . . . inspiration . . . expiration . . . inspiration . . . expiration . . .

"Unknown" No. 2 . . . inspiration . . . expiration . . . inspiration . . . expiration . . . inspiration . . . expiration . . .

"Unknown" No. 3 . . .

"Unknown" No. 4: You are listening to the heart at the apex. Using the bell lightly held, you hear . . . using the bell firmly pressed, you hear . . . using the diaphragm firmly pressed, you hear . . .

"Unknown" No. 5: You are listening to the heart at the apex. Using the bell lightly held, you hear . . . using the bell firmly pressed, you hear . . . using the diaphragm firmly pressed, you hear . . .

CHAPTER 11: FRICTION RUBS—PERICARDIAL AND PLEURAL

Listen now to a pericardial friction rub at the rate of 60 with both systolic and diastolic sounds . . .

Listen to a heart beating 60 times per minute, then only the systolic component of the rub will be added . . .

Listen to a heart beating 60 times per minute, then only the diastolic components of the rub will be added . . .

Now listen to a pericardial friction rub at the heart rate of 120 . . .

Listen to a real heart with a pericardial friction rub. All three components are present . . .

Listen now to a pleural friction rub from a real individual. Note the inspiratory/expiratory components . . .

Compare a pleural friction rub to a pericardial friction rub. First a pleural friction rub . . . now a pericardial friction rub . . .

Self-Learning "Unknown" Heart Sounds—Chapter 11

"Unknown" No. 1: You are listening to the left lateral sternal border. You hear the following sound . . .

"Unknown" No. 2: You are listening to the heart at the apex. You hear the following sound . . .

CHAPTER 12: PROSTHETIC VALVE SOUNDS

Listen now to a patient with a caged-ball valve, the Starr-Edwards . . .

Listen now to a patient with a porcine heart valve in the aortic position . . .

Self-Learning "Unknown" Heart Sounds—Chapter 12

"Unknown" No. 1 . . .

"Unknown" No. 2 . . .

CHAPTER 13: SOUNDS AFTER HEART SURGERY AND OTHER SOUNDS

Listen now to a patient with pericardial friction rub . . .

Listen now to a patient with a paradoxical splitting of the second heart sound as heard with an endocardial pacemaker in the right ventricle . . .

Listen now to a patient with a pericardial knock . . .

Listen now to a patient with a left atrial myxoma . . .

Self-Learning "Unknown" Heart Sounds—Chapter 13

"Unknown" No. 1 . . .

"Unknown" No. 2 . . .

"Unknown" No. 3 . . .
"Unknown" No. 4 . . .

CHAPTER 14: COMMON ADULT ABNORMALITIES

Listen now to the sounds of mitral regurgitation as recorded from a real heart. You are listening at the apex with the bell lightly held. Note the presence of an S_3 . . .

Listen now to the sounds of tricuspid regurgitation as recorded from a real heart. You are listening at the left lateral sternal border with the diaphragm firmly pressed . . .

Listen now to the sounds of aortic stenosis as recorded from a real heart. An aortic ejection sound is heard and then the murmur of aortic stenosis. You are listening at base right . . .

Listen now to the sounds of pulmonic stenosis as recorded from a real heart. A pulmonic ejection sound is first heard and then the murmur of pulmonic stenosis. You are listening at base left . . .

Listen now to the sounds of aortic regurgitation as recorded from a real heart. You are listening at Erb's point with the diaphragm firmly pressed and with the patient leaning forward . . .

Listen now to the sounds of pulmonic regurgitation as recorded from a real heart. You are listening at base left with the diaphragm firmly pressed . . .

Listen now to the sounds of mitral stenosis as recorded from a real heart. You are listening at the apex with the bell lightly held . . .

Listen now to the sounds of tricuspid stenosis as recorded from a real heart. You are listening at the left lateral sternal border with the bell lightly held . . .

Self-Learning "Unknown" Heart Sounds—Chapter 14

"Unknown" No. 1: You are listening to the heart at the apex. The sound radiates toward the left axilla and left sternal border. It may also radiate to base right. Using the diaphragm firmly pressed, you hear . . .

"Unknown" No. 2: You are listening to the heart at base right. The sound radiates bilaterally into the neck and down to the apex. Using either the bell or diaphragm, you hear . . .

CHAPTER 15: GERIATRIC HEART SOUNDS

Listen now to the sounds of aortic sclerosis as recorded from a real heart. You are listening at base right with either the bell or diaphragm . . .

Listen now to the sounds of aortic stenosis as recorded from a real heart. You are listening at base right with either the bell or diaphragm . . .

Listen now to the sounds of mitral regurgitation as recorded from a real heart. You are listening at the apex with the diaphragm firmly pressed. Note the presence of an S_3 . . .

Listen now to the sounds of tricuspid regurgitation as recorded from a real heart. You are listening at the left sternal border with the diaphragm firmly pressed . . .

Listen now to the sounds of mitral stenosis as recorded from a real heart. You are listening at the apex with the bell lightly held . . .

Listen now to the sounds of tricuspid stenosis as recorded from a real heart. You are listening at the left sternal border with the diaphragm firmly pressed . . .

Listen now to the sounds of aortic regurgitation as recorded from a real heart. You are listening at Erb's point with the diaphragm firmly pressed. The patient is leaning forward . . .

Listen now to the sounds of pulmonic regurgitation as recorded from a real heart. You are listening at base left with the diaphragm firmly pressed . . .

Self-Learning "Unknown" Heart Sounds—Chapter 15

"Unknown" No. 1: You are listening to the heart at the apex. The sound also radiates toward the left axilla and left sternal border. It may also radiate to base right. Using the diaphragm firmly pressed, you hear . . .

"Unknown" No. 2: You are listening to the heart at base right. The sound also radiates bilaterally into the neck and down to the apex. Using either the bell or diaphragm, you hear . . .

CHAPTER 16: INTRODUCTION TO PEDIATRIC AUSCULTATION

Listen now to a fetal heart rate of 130 beats per minute. You are listening over the pregnant abdomen with a fetoscope . . .

Listen now to a newborn with a heart rate of 130 beats per minute. You are listening at the apex with the diaphragm firmly pressed . . .

Listen now to an S_3 at a heart rate of 130 beats per minute. You are listening at the apex with the bell lightly held . . .

Listen now to an S_4. You are listening at the apex with the bell lightly held . . .

Listen now to a quadruple rhythm. You are listening at the apex with the bell lightly held . . .

Listen now to a summation gallop. You are listening at the apex with the bell lightly held . . .

Listen now to a physiological split second. Note that the split is heard during inspiration and is not heard during expiration. You are listening at base left with the diaphragm firmly pressed . . .

Listen now to a fixed split S_2. You are listening at base left with the diaphragm firmly pressed . . .

Self-Learning "Unknown" Heart Sounds—Chapter 16

"Unknown" No. 1: You are listening to the heart at base left. Using the diaphragm applied firmly, you hear . . .

"Unknown" No. 2: You are listening to the heart at base left. Using the diaphragm applied firmly, you hear . . .

"Unknown" No. 3: You are listening to the heart at the apex. Using the bell lightly held, you hear . . .

CHAPTER 17: PEDIATRIC SYSTOLIC MURMURS

Listen now to Still's murmur from a real heart. You are listening over the right ventricle between the left lateral sternal border and the apex with either the bell or diaphragm . . .

Listen now to a physiologic systolic ejection murmur from a real heart. You are listening over the left mid to upper sternal border with the diaphragm firmly pressed . . .

Listen now to a pulmonary flow murmur from a real heart. You are listening over base left with either the bell or diaphragm . . .

Listen now to mitral valve prolapse from a real heart. You are listening at the apex with the diaphragm firmly pressed . . .

Listen now to mitral regurgitation from a real heart. You are listening at the apex with the bell lightly held. Note the audible S_3 . . .

Listen now to tricuspid regurgitation from a real heart. You are listening at the apex with the diaphragm firmly pressed . . .

Listen now to aortic stenosis from a real heart. You are listening at base right with the diaphragm firmly pressed . . .

Listen now to pulmonic stenosis from a real heart. You are listening at base right with the diaphragm firmly pressed . . .

Listen now to Eisenmenger syndrome from a real heart. You are listening at base left with the diaphragm firmly pressed . . .

Listen now to tetralogy of Fallot from a real heart. You are listening at the third to fourth left intercostal space with the diaphragm firmly pressed . . .

Listen now to a ventricular septal defect from a real heart. You are listening at the third to fourth left intercostal space with the diaphragm firmly pressed . . .

Self-Learning "Unknown" Heart Sounds—Chapter 17

"Unknown" No. 1: You are listening to a real heart over the right ventricle between the left lateral sternal border and the apex. You hear a systolic murmur which has a groaning, twanging quality. Using either the bell or diaphragm, you hear . . .

"Unknown" No. 2: You are listening to a real heart of a 10-year-old at base right. The harsh murmur radiates to the apex and bilaterally into the neck. Using either the bell or diaphragm, you hear . . .

CHAPTER 18: PEDIATRIC DIASTOLIC MURMURS

Listen now to aortic regurgitation from a real heart. You are listening over Erb's point with the diaphragm firmly pressed. The child is leaning forward . . .

Listen now to the sounds of pulmonic regurgitation as recorded from a real heart. You are listening at base left with the diaphragm firmly pressed . . .

Listen now to mitral stenosis from a real heart. You are listening at the apex with the bell lightly held . . .

Listen now to tricuspid stenosis from a real heart. You are listening at the left lateral sternal border with the bell lightly held . . .

Self-Learning "Unknown" Heart Sounds—Chapter 18

"Unknown" No. 1: You are listening to the heart at the apex. Using the bell lightly held, you hear . . .

"Unknown" No. 2: You are listening to the heart at Erb's point. The child is leaning forward. Using the diaphragm firmly pressed, you hear . . .

CHAPTER 19: PEDIATRIC MURMURS WITH BOTH SYSTOLIC AND DIASTOLIC COMPONENTS

Listen now to an ostium secundum atrial septal defect from a real heart. You are listening along the lower left sternal border with the bell lightly held . . .

Listen now to a cervical venous hum from a real heart. You are listening just above the right clavicle with the bell lightly held . . .

Listen now to a patent ductus arteriosus from a real heart. You are listening at the middle to upper left sternal border with either the bell or diaphragm . . .

Listen now to a large ventricular septal defect from a real heart. You are listening at the third to fourth intercostal space to the left of the sternum with either the bell or diaphragm chest piece . . .

Listen now to the continuous murmur of the Blalock-Taussig shunt from a real heart. You are listening under the clavicle on the side of the shunt and over the operative scar with the diaphragm firmly pressed . . .

Self-Learning "Unknown" Heart Sounds—Chapter 19

"Unknown" No. 1: You are listening to a real heart above the right clavicle. Using the bell lightly held, you hear . . .

"Unknown" No. 2: You are listening to a real heart at the middle to upper left sternal border. Using either the bell or diaphragm, you hear . . .

Bibliography

Beers MH, Berkow R, Editors: *The Merck manual of geriatrics.* ed 3, Whitehouse Station, NJ, 2000, Merck Research Laboratories.

Behrman RE, Kliegman RM, Jenson HB: *Nelson textbook of pediatrics,* ed16, Philadelphia, 2000, WB Saunders.

Caccamo L, Erickson B: *Cardiac auscultation,* Youngstown, 1975, St. Elizabeth Hospital Medical Center.

Erickson B: Detecting abnormal heart sounds, *Nurs 86* 16(1):58-63, 1986.

Erickson RL: An in vitro study of mechanical heart valve sound loudness, *J Heart Valve Dis* 3(3):330-334, 1994.

Frankl WS, Brest AN: *Valvular heart disease: comprehensive evaluation and treatment, cardiovascular clinics,* ed 2, Philadelphia, 1993, FA Davis.

Harvey WP, Canfield DC: *Clinical auscultation of the cardiovascular system: tapes with companion tests,* Newton, NJ, 1989, Laënnec Publishing.

Lerner Research Institute: *A heart valve tutorial,* website: http://www.lerner.ccf.org/bme/valve/tutorial/

Moody LY: Pediatric cardiovascular assessment and referral in the primary care setting, *Nurse Pract* 22(1):120,123-126,128-129, 1997.

Pelech AN: The cardiac murmur when to refer? *Pediatr Clin North Am* 45(1): 107-122, 1998.

Rush Children's Heart Center: Innocent heart murmurs, website: http://www.rchc.rush.edu/rmawebfiles/htmurmurs.htm.

Tallis R, Fillit H, Brocklehurst JC: *Brocklehurst's textbook of geriatric medicine and gerontology,* ed 5, New York, 1998, Churchill Livingstone.

Vaska PL: Sternal wound infections, *AACN Clin Issues* 4(3):475-483, 1993.

Wong DL et al: *Whaley & Wong's nursing care of infants and children,* ed 6, St Louis, 1999, Mosby.

Glossary

A

A₂: Aortic component of the second heart sound (S_2); normally comes before the pulmonic component (P_2).

Allograft: Tissue graft from individual of the same species (isograft).

Aortic ejection sound: See Ejection sounds, Aortic.

Aortic regurgitation or aortic valve regurgitation: Inability of the aortic valve to close completely, permitting backflow of blood from the aorta into the left ventricle. It may be caused by congenital or acquired disease.

Aortic sclerosis or aortic valve sclerosis: Results from degenerative fibrous thickening and stiffening of the base of the aortic cusps as they insert into the sinuses of Valsalva. This occurs without commissural fusion, without impairment of cusp mobility, and accordingly without obstruction.

Aortic stenosis or aortic valve sclerosis: Inability of the aortic valve to open completely, restricting blood flow from the left ventricle out into the aorta. A congenital bicuspid valve is often the cause but it may also be acquired.

Aortic valve: Semilunar valve that prevents the backflow of blood from the aorta into the left ventricle during ventricular diastole. The closure of this valve is responsible for the first component (A_2) of the second heart sound.

Apex: Area of cardiac auscultation that is also known as the *point of maximum impulse* (*PMI*) of the heart against the chest wall. In the normal adult it is at the fifth intercostal space (ICS) to the left of the sternum at the midclavicular line. Sounds from the mitral valve and the left heart are heard best in this area. In the child, the PMI changes with advancing age. It is at the level of the fourth ICS until age 7 years, when it drops to the fifth ICS.

Arterial supraclavicular bruit: Innocent sound that is attributed to turbulence at the origins of the brachiocephalic vessels.

Atrial kick: Slang term for atrial systole or atrial contraction that may contribute 20% to 25% to ventricular filling. It occurs during the late filling phase of the ventricular diastolic period but only if atrial contraction occurs. It can never occur in the presence of atrial fibrillation.

Atrial septal defect (ASD): Congenital cardiac anomaly characterized by an abnormal opening between the two atria. Of all congenital heart diseases seen in infancy, 10% to 15% are ASDs. Females are more commonly affected than are males. The three types of ASDs are (1) ostium primum, which is a congenital opening in the septum near the atrial-ventricular (AV) valve and associated with a cleft mitral valve leaflet; (2) ostium secundum, which is a congenital defect at the fossa ovalis; and (3) sinus venosus, which is a defect posterior to fossa ovalis and associated with partial anomalous pulmonary return.

Atrial systole: See Systole, atrial.

Auscultogram: Graphic method of charting heart sounds.

B

Base left: Area of cardiac auscultation; the second intercostal space to the left of the sternum. Sounds from the pulmonic valve are heard best in this area.

Base right: Area of cardiac auscultation; the second intercostal space to the right of the sternum. Sounds from the aortic valve are heard best in this area.

Bell chestpiece: Component of the stethoscope that has a shallow shell with a diameter as large as feasible to permit an air seal when held lightly on the chest wall (leaving no after-imprint). It transmits sounds of *low* frequency.

Bicuspid aortic valve: Congenital deformity of the aortic valve that has only two functional leaflets instead of the normal three.

Bileaflet: Type of mechanical prosthetic heart valve with two semicircular leaflets mounted on a circular sewing ring that opens in the center.

Biologic prosthetic heart valve: Valve made from tissue of the same species (allograft) or from different species (xenograft).

Blalock-Taussig operation: Surgical construction of a shunt as a temporary measure to overcome congenital pulmonary stenosis and atrial septal defect. It creates an end-to-side subclavian-artery to pulmonary-artery shunt.

Bovine pericardial heart valve: Prosthetic heart valve made from a cow. It consists of three identical cusps mounted on a cloth-covered frame.

C

Caged-ball: Type of mechanical prosthetic heart valve consisting of a ball that moves freely within a three- or four-sided metallic cage mounted on a circular sewing ring.

Cardiac cycle: Period from the beginning of one beat of the heart to the beginning of the next succeeding beat; consists of two phases: one of contraction, *systole*—atrial and ventricular; and one of relaxation, *diastole*—atrial and ventricular.

Cervical venous hum: Innocent sound produced by turbulence in blood flow in the internal jugular vein as blood flows from the head and neck into the thorax.

Click: High frequency sound that is heard after the first heart sound (S_1). It may be a single or multiple sound(s) heard in the middle of the ventricular systolic period; often associated with mitral valve prolapse.

Compliance: Ratio of change in volume to a change in pressure (V/P). Ventricular compliance is decreased in the presence of any condition that limits the ability of the ventricle(s) to expand. Decreased ventricular compliance is one mechanism responsible for the production of the third (S_3) and the fourth (S_4) heart sounds.

D

Diaphragm chestpiece: Component of the stethoscope that has a taut (stiff) material drawn across its diameter. When it is firmly applied to the chest wall (leaving an after-imprint), it transmits sounds of *high* frequency.

Diastole, ventricular: Period of ventricular filling that follows closure of the aortic and pulmonic valves. The ventricular diastolic period is divided into three phases:
1. First third of the diastolic period, which has two subdivisions—the isovolumic relaxation phase and the rapid filling phase.
2. Middle third of the diastolic period, during which both atria and ventricles are relaxed.
3. Last third of diastole, or the late filling phase, during which atrial contraction takes place.

Diastolic murmurs: See Murmurs, Diastolic.

Duration: Length of time that a sound lasts. Normal heart sounds (S_1 and S_2) are of short duration. Cardiac murmurs or rubs are of long duration.

E

Eisenmenger's syndrome: Name loosely applied to any condition with a left-to-right shunt, such as atrial septal defect (ASD), ventricular septal defect (VSD), and persistent ductus arteriosus, that subsequently develops severe pulmonary vascular hypertension.

Ejection murmur: See Murmurs—Mid.

Ejection sounds: High frequency "clicking" sounds occurring very shortly after the first sound. They may be of either aortic or pulmonic origin.

Aortic: High frequency "clicking" sound heard best at the apex but may be heard anywhere on a straight line from base right to the apex. Heard in valvular aortic stenosis, aortic insufficiency, coarctation of the aorta, and aneurysm of the ascending aorta.

Pulmonic: High-frequency "clicking" sound heard best at base left but may be heard anywhere along the left lateral sternal border. It may be heard in pulmonic stenosis, pulmonary hypertension, atrial septal defect, pulmonary embolism, or hyperthyroidism or in conditions causing enlargement of the pulmonary artery.

F

Fetal heart sound: Sounds from the fetal heart heard through the maternal abdomen in pregnancy.

First heart sound (S_1): Initial sound heard—also known as S_1. It occurs at the beginning of ventricular systole when ventricular volume is maximal. It is a result of the closure of the mitral (M_1) and tricuspid (T_1) valves.

 Split, normal: When both mitral and tricuspid closure are distinguishable and are 0.02 second apart.

 Split, wide: Mitral and tricuspid closure sounds occur wider apart from either electrical or mechanical causes that result in ventricular asynchrony.

Fourth heart sound (S_4): Low frequency sound heard just before the first heart sound. It is a result of decreased ventricular compliance or increased volume of filling. It also is known as *atrial gallop, presystolic gallop, S_4 gallop,* and S_4.

Frequency: Number of wave cycles generated per second by a vibrating body. It is the vibratory movement of an object in motion that initiates the sound wave cycles that can be discerned with the stethoscope.

 High: The greater the number of wave cycles per second generated by a vibrating body, the higher the frequency. Sounds of high frequency are heard best with the diaphragm chestpiece firmly pressed.

 Low: The fewer the number of wave cycles per second generated by a vibrating body, the lower the frequency. Sounds of low frequency are heard best with the bell chestpiece lightly applied.

 Mid: Combination of high and low frequencies. Sound heard equally well with either bell or diaphragm.

H

Heart sound simulator: Electronic device designed to generate all normal and abnormal heart sound patterns by the independent variation of all sound parameters.

Heterologous: Derived from tissue of a different species (xenograft).

I

Innocent murmurs: See Murmurs, Innocent.

Intensity: Determines the loudness of the perceived sound. It is related to the height of the sound wave produced by a vibrating object. Objects vibrating with great energy are heard as loud sounds. Objects vibrating with low energy are heard as soft sounds.

Intraaortic balloon pump: Mechanical device that aids the heart's circulation through counterpulsation; it expands in diastole and collapses in systole.

Isograft: Tissue grafts from individuals of the same species (allograft).

Isovolumic contraction: Phase during the first part of ventricular systole. It begins with the first initial rise in ventricular pressure after the closure of the mitral and tricuspid valves.

Isovolumic relaxation: Phase during the first third of the ventricular diastole. Initially in this period, no blood is entering the ventricles and the ventricles therefore are not increasing in volume.

L

Late filling phase: Phase during the last third of ventricular diastole. It is at this time that the atrial kick or atrial contraction takes place.

Left lateral recumbent: Position for cardiac auscultation in which the patient is lying on his or her left side with left arm extended under head. The heart is brought closer to the chest wall in this position. Also, the exertion of turning to this position increases heart rate. This position may be useful in making audible the diastolic rumble of mitral stenosis or the low frequency third heart sound (S_3) of congestive heart failure.

Left lateral sternal border (LLSB): Area of cardiac auscultation that is at the left fourth intercostal space to the left of the sternum. Sounds from the tricuspid valve and right heart are heard best in this area.

M

M_1: Mitral component of the first heart sound. This is normally the first component and occurs just after the mitral valve closes; normally comes before the tricuspid component (T_1).

Mammary soufflé: Innocent murmur that may be heard in the latter months of pregnancy or during lactation. It seems to be caused by increased blood flow in the internal mammary and intercostal arteries.

Mechanical prosthetic heart valve: Type of prosthetic heart valve made from a combination of metal alloys, pyrolytic carbon, and Dacron.

Mediastinal crunch: Presence of air in the mediastinum that produces a series of scratchy sounds.

Mitral regurgitation or mitral valve regurgitation: Inability of the mitral valve to close completely, permitting backflow of blood from the left ventricle into the left atrium. It may be caused by either congenital or acquired disease. It is also known as *mitral incompetence* or *mitral insufficiency.*

Mitral stenosis or mitral valve stenosis: Inability of the mitral valve to open completely, restricting blood flow from the left atrium to the left ventricle. Rheumatic fever is a common cause.

Mitral valve: Bicuspid valve between the left atrium and the left ventricle; one of two "A-V" valves; prevents backflow of blood from left ventricle to left atrium during ventricular systole. Closure of this valve is responsible for the first component (M_1) of the first heart sound.

Mitral valve prolapse: Syndrome associated with a midsystolic click and a late systolic murmur. One of the mitral leaflets, usually the posterior one, balloons into the left atrium at the point of maximal ventricular ejection. The click is heard when the chordae tendineae suddenly stop the ballooning leaflet. If the leaflets pull apart, a late systolic murmur of mitral regurgitation also may be heard. Also known as *Barlow's syndrome, floppy mitral valve,* or *click-murmur syndrome.*

Murmurs: Sustained noises that are audible during the time periods of systole, diastole, or both.

Continuous murmur: Sustained noise that begins in systole and continues through the second heart sound into all or part of diastole.

Diastolic murmurs: Sustained noises that are audible between the second heart sound and the next first heart sound. They should be considered organic and not normal. Common causes include mitral or tricuspid valve stenosis and aortic or pulmonic valve regurgitation.

Early: Peaks in the first third of the cycle.

Innocent: Benign or functional sustained noise that is caused by a normal degree of turbulence as blood moves from one area to another. This turbulence sets the surrounding tissues into vibration, which is transmitted out through the chest and to the stethoscope.

Late: Peaks in the last third of the cycle.

Mid: Peaks in the middle of the cycle; "crescendo/decrescendo" (diamond shaped). Also known as *ejection murmur.*

Pan: Heard continuously throughout the cycle.

Systolic murmurs: Sustained noises that are audible between the first and the second heart sounds. Common causes include mitral or tricuspid valve regurgitation and aortic or pulmonic valve stenosis.

Myxoma: Soft tumor composed primarily of connective tissue.

O

Opening snap: Short, high-frequency "click" or "snap" that occurs after the second heart sound. It is most often produced by the opening of a stenosed, thickened, or distorted mitral or tricuspid valve.

Ostium primum atrial septal defect (ASD): Congenital opening in the septum near the A-V valve and associated with a cleft mitral valve leaflet.

Ostium secundum atrial septal defect (ASD): Congenital defect at the fossa ovalis.

P

P$_2$: Pulmonic component of the second heart sound; usually follows aortic component (A$_2$).

Pacemaker: Electrical apparatus used to electrically stimulate the heart and regulate the heartbeat.

Patent ductus arteriosus (PDA): Results when the functional closure of the ductus arteriosus fails to occur at birth. In fetal life the ductus arteriosus connects the pulmonary artery to the aorta and shunts oxygenated blood directly into the systemic circulation, bypassing the lungs. Normal closure occurs a few hours after birth although complete closure may take several weeks.

Pericardial knock: Early diastolic sound occurring in constrictive pericarditis.

Physiologic systolic ejection murmur: Innocent murmur caused by flow of blood as it is ejected from the left ventricle.

Pitch: Subjective sensation that indicates to the listener whether the tone is high or low on a musical scale.

Point of maximal impulse (PMI): See Apex.

Porcine heart valve: Prosthetic heart valve made from a pig. It is mounted on a semiflexible stent and preserved with glutaraldehyde.

Prosthetic heart valve: Artificial valve, either mechanical or biological, used to replace a damaged heart valve.

Pulmonary flow murmur: Innocent murmur of infancy that results from turbulence caused by changes in systolic pressure from the pulmonary trunk to its branches. It disappears, usually within a few months, as the infant grows.

Pulmonic ejection sound: See Ejection sounds, Pulmonic.

Pulmonic regurgitation or pulmonic valve regurgitation: Inability of the pulmonary valve to close completely, permitting backflow of blood from the pulmonary artery into the right ventricle. It is not a commonly acquired adult pathologic condition and is most often a congenital defect.

Pulmonic stenosis or pulmonic valve stenosis: Inability of the pulmonary valve to open completely, restricting blood flow from the right ventricle to the pulmonary artery. Its cause is most commonly congenital although it may be acquired.

Pulmonic valve: Semilunar valve that prevents backflow of blood from the pulmonary artery into the right ventricle during ventricular diastole. Closure of the valve is responsible for the second component (P$_2$) of the second heart sound.

Q

Quality: Sound characteristic that distinguishes two sounds that have equal degrees of frequency and intensity but come from a different source—e.g., piano from violin, or heart from lung.

Blowing: Mainly high frequency.

Harsh: Mix of high and low frequencies—slightly more high than low.

Rough: Mix of high and low frequencies—slightly more low than high.

Rumble: Mainly low frequency.

R

Rapid filling phase: Phase during the first third of ventricular diastole. It occurs when ventricular pressure is less than atrial pressure. The mitral and tricuspid valves then open, and blood rapidly enters the ventricles.

Rapid ventricular ejection: Phase during the first part of ventricular systole. It follows the isovolumic contraction phase. It occurs when ventricular pressure exceeds the pressure in the aorta and the pulmonary artery, forcing the aortic and pulmonic valves open and causing blood to be rapidly ejected from the ventricles.

S

S_1: See First heart sound.

S_2: See Second heart sound.

S_3: See Third heart sound.

S_4: See Fourth heart sound.

Second heart sound (S_2): Second sound heard in a normal heart—also known as S_2. It occurs at the end of ventricular systole. It is a result of the closure of the aortic (A_2) and pulmonic (P_2) valves.

Split, fixed: Does not change its width with inspiration or expiration.

Split, narrow: Aortic (A_2) and pulmonic (P_2) components are closer together than normal—<0.03 second. The split is heard on *inspiration* and is single on expiration.

Split, paradoxical: Reversal of the normal closure sequence of S_2, with pulmonic closure (P_2) occurring before aortic closure (A_2). This split is heard during *expiration* and becomes single on inspiration, which is the opposite of a normal or physiological split.

Split, physiological: Aortic (A_2) and pulmonic (P_2) components that make up the second sound are separately distinguishable—0.03 second apart. The split is heard on *inspiration* and is single on expiration.

Split, wide: Delay in pulmonic valve closure can cause the physiological split to be accentuated or increased—0.04 to 0.05 second. The split is heard during *inspiration* and becomes single on expiration.

Sine wave: Up and down or to and fro undulating or wavy line.

Sinus venosus atrial septal defect (ASD): Defect posterior to fossa ovalis and associated with partial anomalous pulmonary return.

Split: When both components that make up a sound are separately distinguishable, the sound is said to "split." Duration of 0.02 second between the sounds is necessary for the ear to be able to make this distinction. See First heart sound, Split; and Second heart sound, Split.

Sternum, unstable: Indicative of sternal dehiscence after a median sternotomy. Sternal click is a sign of instability.

Stethoscope: Acoustical instrument that uses the vibration of sounds reacting on the air column enclosed in tubing to transmit sounds to the listener's ear. When used for heart sounds, a chestpiece that permits differentiation between low and high frequency sounds (traditionally the bell and diaphragm) is necessary.

Still's murmur: Innocent murmur that originates from periodic vibrations of pulmonic leaflets at their attachments. It was first described by Dr. Still in 1909.

Subcutaneous emphysema: Presence of air or gas in the subcutaneous tissues.

Systole, atrial: Period in cardiac cycle. It occurs during the last third of ventricular diastole or during the late filling phase. During this period, contraction of the atrium takes place and the remaining blood is squeezed from the atrium. This is known also as the *atrial kick*. Atrial systole may contribute 20% to 25% to ventricular filling. The contribution is less at faster heart rates—more than 100 beats/minute.

Systole, ventricular: Period in cardiac cycle. It follows closure of the mitral and tricuspid valves. This systolic period is divided into two phases. The first phase includes the isovolumic contraction phase and the rapid ventricular ejection phase. During the second phase, which occurs to the latter part of ventricular systole, ventricular pressure falls and reduced ventricular ejection occurs. This period lasts until ventricular ejection stops and ventricular diastole begins.

Systolic murmurs: See Murmurs, Systolic.

T

T_1:   Second component of the first sound. It normally occurs after M_1 (the mitral component) just after the tricuspid valve closes.

Tetralogy of Fallot: Most common congenital lesion that produces cyanosis. In this pathologic condition, there are various degrees of (1) pulmonary valvular stenosis, or infundibular stenosis, that result in decreased pulmonary blood flow; (2) a ventricular septal defect (VSD) with a right-to-left shunt; (3) an aorta that overrides the VSD; and (4) right ventricular hypertrophy.

Third heart sound (S_3):   Low frequency sound heard just after the second heart sound. It is a diastolic sound that occurs during the early rapid filling phase of ventricular diastole. It is a result of decreased ventricular compliance or increased ventricular diastolic volume. It also is known as a *ventricular gallop, protodiastolic gallop, S_3 gallop,* or S_3.

Thrill: Continuous palpable sensation felt on the precordium. It is comparable to the vibration felt when a cat purrs.

Thrust: Palpable (sometimes even visible) intermittent sensation. This is the sensation felt when palpating the point of maximal impulse (PMI) at the apex of the heart.

Tilting disk: Type of mechanical valve with a free-floating, lens-shaped disk mounted on a circular sewing ring.

Timing: Determining whether sound is occurring during the systolic or diastolic period.

Timing, finer: Determining whether sound is occurring early, mid, late, or pan in the systolic or diastolic period.

Tricuspid regurgitation or tricuspid valve regurgitation: Inability of the tricuspid valve to close completely, permitting backflow of blood from the right ventricle into the right atrium.

Tricuspid stenosis or tricuspid valve stenosis: Inability of the tricuspid valve to open completely, restricting blood flow from the right atrium to the right ventricle.

Tricuspid valve: Three-leaflet valve between the right atrium and the right ventricle: one of two atrial-ventricular (A-V) valves; prevents backflow of blood from the right ventricle to right atrium during ventricular systole. Closure of this valve is responsible for the second component (T_1) of the first heart sound.

Turbulence: Smooth blood flow is disturbed, and the blood flows crosswise in the vessel or chamber, as well as along the vessel. This causes eddy currents similar to a whirlpool and produces vibrations that are audible.

V

Ventricular diastole: See Diastole, ventricular.

Ventricular septal defect (VSD): Congenital defect that results from a hole in the ventricular septum. It is the most common pathologic condition associated with a systolic murmur in children. The direction of blood flow through the defect depends on the degree of pulmonary vascular outflow obstruction from either pulmonary stenosis or pulmonary hypertension. When this pulmonary outflow resistance is low, the flow is left to right; when this resistance is high, the flow is right to left.

Ventricular systole: See Systole, ventricular.

X

Xenograft: Derived from tissue of a different species (heterologous).

Index